C WALK HOME
Love, Cancer, and the Agony of Letting Go

Jennifer Sanfilippo

ROCHESTER, NEW YORK

Copyright © 2023 by **Jennifer Sanfilippo**

All rights reserved. No part of this publication may be reproduced, distributed or transmitted in any form or by any means, without prior written permission.

Jennifer Sanfilippo Consulting, LLC
Rochester, New York
www.jennifer-sanfilippo.com

Publisher's Note: The stories in this book reflect the author's recollection of events. Some names, locations, and identifying characteristics have been changed to protect the privacy of those depicted. Dialogue has been re-created from memory.

Book Layout © 2023

Cover Art © James P. Barbero
Cover Design © Giacomo R. Barbero
Cover Design Consultant © Gianni S. Barbero

Our Last Walk Home: Love, Cancer, and the Agony of Letting Go/ Jennifer Sanfilippo. -- 1st ed.
ISBN 979-8-9900311-0-4

In loving memory of my husband, Jim.
This is to say that you will always matter to me.

To my greatest inspirations and sources of joy,
Giacomo and Gianni.

I love you all more than words can say.

CONTENTS

Preface i
Prologue i
The End 1
The Emergency Room 15
Everyone Equals No One 25
From Worse to Worser 31
Violated 45
Forty Days in the Hole 59
Hospital Life 65
Settling in 75
Friends and Family 89
    Our sons 94
    The family area 98
The "Lay" of the Land 103
Treatment 109
February 117
Home Again, Home Again, Jiggety-Jig 129
Covid Creep 139
    The community pool 147
    Fever 149
    No retreat, no surrender 152
See-Saw Margery Daw 155
Psychosocial Support 163
Zero Minus Five 171

Making love 175
Paddling a Leaky Boat 179
    The caper 185
    The ants go marching in 188
Shock and Awe 191
    On a hot summer night 196
Déjà Vu 207
    Making meaning 217
    Welcome to our shit show 222
The Dimming of the Day 229
    The thinking light 231
Epilogue 235
Acknowledgements 239

Preface

I'm wearing one of Jim's sweaters as I sit in our bedroom beneath our wedding photo, three feet away from our bed. The bed where Jim took his last breath. I am so upset with myself because I washed all of his clothes before I knew he was going to die. I often find myself in Jim's closet, hugging his clothes, going from shirt to shirt, sniffing like a bloodhound. Catching a whiff of him gives me a moment in heaven. I close my eyes and hold my breath, suspending his essence in the back of my nose. I try to keep it there as long as I can. For a split second, it's like he's there with me.

With each passing day, I become increasingly obsessed with the idea that I need to shape a lasting record of the course of our lives from January through July, 2020. But every time I try to write, my thoughts scatter like cockroaches in abrupt light. The only difference is my thoughts don't hide. They scramble around all haywire in a confined space. The mental activity shorts my circuits. I can think of so many things to say, but by the time I try to write, I'm paralyzed. All I can do is stare. At anything. Anywhere. Out the window. At the ceiling. My eyes fix, allowing my thoughts to slow down and walk the inner void of my soul. When I snap out of it, I either clean something, cook something or take care of an animal.

Jim's cancer took him so fucking fast! I'm desperate to understand what the hell happened, so I turn to collecting every single artifact from those days and studying each of them like a research scientist. I spend hours reading Jim's medical records and comparing them to my notes and CaringBridge posts. Alternately, I look at photos and listen to music, bathing my soul in my memories of Jim. It's agony to see him—to see us—in all our lovely life together. Smiling, laughing, making things, doing things. Loving each other, our kids, our friends and families. By the time I pull myself away, I'm in despair. Yet I press forward, reliving the brutality of Jim's last six months. Piece by piece, I stitch together the evidence of Jim's existence with the audacity of that Modern Prometheus, Dr. Frankenstein, in an attempt to breathe life back into him—an act of defiance as well as love. I delve into this obsession with reincarnation like a crazed sorceress.

But is it so farfetched to believe that memorializing Jim's life in story form will leave an indelible mark on the hearts of all who read it? Thereby keeping him alive in perpetuity?

And so it goes: *Our Last Walk Home* is a story about family viewed from behind the plexiglass of a cancer diagnosis. You're invited to read our story and share this tale with anyone who wants to know what our battle was like. With anyone who wants to view the inside of a tenacious marriage. With anyone who wants to help me hold on to the memories of my exceptional husband Jim.

Prologue

If you live in a climate that makes a big production of wintry weather, the sound of someone trying to get their car dislodged from a snow bank is unmistakable. *Rindidadida. Riiiiiinndidadida. Riiiiiiiinnndidadidadida.*

Most folks who grow up in a snowy region are familiar with the rocking method employed to extricate a car from the snow. It doesn't always work, mind you, but the knowledge is crucial to giving yourself a fighting chance. You need at least two people, one person pushing while the driver is working the gas pedal. There is no gunning of the engine, which is what most people inexperienced with snow and ice are wont to do. Gunning it and hoping for the best is what digs you in deeper, eventually cementing your car in place until spring.

Rocking the car is a nuanced choreography in which the participants have to be completely in sync with each other. It's notable that, in my neighborhood, where street parking is the norm, this dance is often done between total strangers.

Let's say we need to get the car moving forward. First, the driver puts the car in drive while the other person (or people, depending on the "stuckness" and availability of bodies) stands behind the car. The driver touches the gas lightly, and whoever is in back of the car simultaneously pushes forward. The purpose of the initial effort is not to dislodge the car. The people in back are merely trying to leverage the car's momentum. It's a little bit like pushing a kid on a swing. You don't want to push the little tyke off their perch. You just want to enhance their own pumping power. After the first hit of gas and subsequent push, the car will roll back. The collaborators quickly repeat the process to start a rocking motion. Gas forward, helpers push, car rocks back. Gas forward, people push, car rocks back a little more with momentum. If all goes well, you'll be able to feel the tires gaining traction, and it'll only take a couple more repetitions of the sequence before the driver can accelerate in earnest and the people pushing can put their all into freeing the vehicle. Successful efforts are marked by a heap of patience and collaboration.

The other day I heard the unmistakable sound of a neighbor trying to free their car without the aforementioned game plan. From my window I could see the tires smoking as they ground down into snow and ice while the driver jammed the gas. It wasn't long before the unmistakable sound of rubber hitting asphalt rang out through the whole neighborhood with a *Shcreeeeee! Well now you've done it,* I thought.

It all starts easily enough. Novice drivers or people unfamiliar with snowbelt territory jump into their vehicles as if it were a summer day and plan to drive off to do whatever needs doing. They don't stop to consider the possibility that they might not be able to get out of the four feet of snow the city plows dumped around their car. After their first attempt at an exit is thwarted by the cement-like wall around them, their next thought isn't based in logic. It's more under the umbrella of denial. The fact that they can't easily drive away messes with their head. "I need to go somewhere important! If I don't leave now, I'm going to be late. I'm the master of my destiny and my car works in service of my busy-ness." From that perspective, it makes sense that hitting the gas and *willing* the car forward is their "go to" response. And so they dig in further. It's unfathomable to them that this situation, if not managed carefully, will be the catalyst of an aggravating domino effect, knocking down all their plans for the day.

That's what it was like when we went to the hospital. Both Jim and I were going our usual thousand miles an hour. Large and in charge of our full lives. Sitting in the emergency room for seven hours only aggravated our resolve to keep our frenetic pace. We were fully expecting to get a manageable diagnosis with instructions to "call the doctor in the morning." I could feel my right foot pressing an imaginary gas pedal.

When they told us Jim had cancer and that we had to check in to the cancer center immediately, it wasn't registering with me. I was still gunning the engine. "Can't we go home and call our doctor?" The head of the ER tried not to scream "NO" in my face. She explained that they *strongly* recommended that we go *directly* to the cancer center for *immediate* admission. Okay. Well, I guess maybe this situation is more complicated than we thought.

We were taken upstairs to the cancer center shortly after nine p.m. Our dominoes for the day had all fallen down. What we didn't know at the time was that all our dominoes were about to be taken away for the rest of our lives. My head was like an echo chamber holding these bouncing thoughts: *Three days ago Jim was going about his regular routine. He went to work and went for a run at lunchtime. Saturday night he picked me up from the airport and on our car ride home we planned our next trip together. Sunday morning, he helped friends move furniture. We're both healthy people. We've been active our whole lives. Jim is a force of nature. He's a musician and a visual artist, he has an engaging job, he rebuilt EVERYTHING in our house. In fact, he just single-handedly remodeled our* kitchen. Our college-aged kids are almost out of the house! We're planning the back nine of our employment years to set up for retirement!

Riiiinndidadida. Riiiiinnndidadidadida. Schreeeeeeeeeee!!!!

"Your car isn't going anywhere Ma'am. You're going to have to cancel your plans for today, tomorrow, and, well, the foreseeable future, so STOP GUNNING IT!"

CHAPTER ONE

The End

Activity radiates from the pages of our 2019 family calendar like crackling electricity. Work, school, gigs, trips, hikes and holidays, "Life! Life! Life!" shouts my calendar with a seemingly unstoppable surge of energy.

We had such a fun year. I was laid off at the end of 2018. Greatest 50th birthday present I could ever have received. Though the banking industry just spat me out like expired lunch meat, my eight-year tour of duty had been quite lucrative. Instead of jumping back into the job market, I decided to take a self-funded sabbatical. I had ideas I wanted to explore, so I spent the year writing, taking courses, and producing my own podcast. Unlike my years of work-related travel, my educational pursuits were all conducted from the comfort of my home. I had worked my ass off for years. After running in the rat race like an ultra-marathoner, staying home and taking a load off felt awesome.

Most weekday mornings, I would sit and drink coffee with Josh, our neighborhood Canadian, while Jim got ready for work. Jim and Josh carpooled together, so Josh walked to our house every morning to meet him for their commute. We hung out so often, he became another brother to us. Jim was seldom ready when Josh arrived, so we'd discuss news of the day over breakfast while Jim ran around the house like a chicken with his head cut off. My mental picture of Jim's frantic weekday routine juxtaposed to mine and Josh's coffee house vibe still makes me laugh. Once they finally got out the door, I would go up to my office and work on my projects.

Both of our sons were on the runway to independence. Soon they would be out of the house entirely, leaving us to enjoy our couplehood without distraction. Jim and I were getting to that sweet spot in a marriage, the empty-nester era where we could enjoy each other's company and the quiet beauty of our home like we did pre-kids.

We got in the habit of taking a passeggiata every evening. The seasons would change around us as we walked around the neighborhood and talked about our plans for the future. I was ready for a life transition, admittedly a little bit ahead of Jim. My vision was to launch a remote consulting business so we could travel to warm locales during the winters, providing the opportunity to scout out retirement options. There were so many places we wanted to see.

We already had a couple big trips under our belt that year. The best one by far was an epic hiking trip to search for Forest Fenn's treasure in honor of our 25th wedding anniversary. The search had been on my list of "things to do" since Fenn announced he'd buried the treasure 10 years prior. Now was our big chance! We packed up and went to Wyoming to try our hand at the most fascinating treasure hunt of modern times. We didn't find the treasure, but we did have the trip of our lives.

This fantastic year was capped off by a great Christmas. "Great Christmas" are not words that pass my lips often. I've never been a fan of the holiday. So much so that for the last ten years, I've been on a campaign, albeit unsuccessful, to turn Christmas into Second Thanksgiving, where we could enjoy our families' company without the insanity of inflexible traditions infused with borderline psychotic commercialism.

Jim on the other hand always loved Christmas. He was more excited about the holiday than your typical four-year-old. I remember when we first started dating. We went out with my sister for a few drinks the night before he went home to Rochester for the holidays. As he was leaving my apartment, he turned to us with a huge grin on his face and with a sweeping hand gesture, announced he was going home for some bacala! Soon after, I learned that Jim's family observed the seven fishes tradition. Essentially, on Christmas Eve, you eat seven different fish dishes. Then, at midnight you eat sausage. To this day, I don't understand how stuffing your face with seafood for eight hours, then capping it all off with a block of meat relates to the birth of Jesus. In my mind, gluttony doesn't seem to jive with the call for peace on earth and goodwill to men.

Shortly after we moved in together, it became crystal clear that Jim's staunch family tradition was uncompromising. The slightest hint of a modification was met with stone cold resistance. My family's tradition was very different. My parents had five kids within six years. By the time I was in elementary school, both my parents were working full time as teachers and my dad had an additional part-time job to make ends meet. The pressure around the holidays must have been unbearable. In the early '70s, they were struggling with the dictates of traditional gender roles. That tension bubbled over into unrealistic expectations about domestic duties related to cooking, Christmas shopping, decorating, and all the other trappings that accompany the holiday. Add to that stress stew: my grandparents. The keepers of family social and moral codes placed unreasonable expectations on our family for religious observances and party attendance on Christmas Eve and Christmas Day. Neither side cut anyone a break. The pressure cooker that was Christmas invariably blew up into a spectacular argument between my parents on Christmas Eve. Norman Lear once said his family lived at the edge of their nerves and the top of their lungs. That most certainly described our clan. This was the Christmas tradition I grew up with.

By the time our kids were two and three, I was way over Jim's family tradition. Staying at someone else's house until midnight with little kids while you still had Santa stuff to do was torture. During those years, I asked Jim if there was any possibility that we could skip it. Once. Just once, I would've liked to have stayed home for Christmas. "My parents are older. I don't know how many more Christmases we'll have together," was his reply. Twenty-seven. In case you were wondering. Honestly? My best Christmas in the early days of parenthood happened when the kids were sick, because projectile vomiting qualified as an authorized excuse to stay home.

As a married person, you can be as "over it" as you want, but you still have to find a way to navigate through points of contention. My way was to be angry and bitter about it until February. It helped that my mom didn't pressure us to come over on Christmas Day. Likely still stinging from years of annual Christmas fights, she knew that as a new mom I was under enough pressure. I'm sure she didn't want to see the perpetuation of the Sanfilippo family tradition in my household any more than I did. Old habits die hard though. When the kids were babes, I did a fair amount of Christmas Sanfilippo-style. But one of the great things about being human is that we have the ability to learn from our mistakes and to make different choices. Recognizing that I needed to wield compromise like a cudgel to bash the shackles of my old habits, I eventually learned how to set boundaries and create our own holiday traditions. Though Jim was firm on his Christmas Eve fish-fest, he was open to everything else I wanted to do on the other days. It took some practice, but with a lot of patience and shared purpose we were able to carve out our own peace on earth.

Then, the moment I'd been waiting for! Christmas 2019, Jim's 89-year-old mom announced she would no longer host Christmas Eve! *Hallelujah!* I thought. *Christmas Eve at home! We can relax! Build a fire and sit in front of the tree! We finally get a Christmas Eve at home together!* The warm glow of my Christmas Eve fantasy was interrupted by Jim's announcement that he had booked a gig for that night. No fucking joke. The first free Christmas Eve in 27 years and my husband booked a gig. I'm going to let you imagine how that conversation went.

Fortunately, turning 50, coupled with the joys of unemployment had mellowed me out considerably. I turned my focus to Christmas Day. We were hosting my whole family. Eighteen high-energy personalities. Jim and I collaborated on all aspects of the festivities. We had been watching a lot of cooking shows on public television. Steve Raichlen in particular enticed us with his smoked meats and barbecues. We decided on one of his recipes for ribs and pulled pork instead of our regular labor-intensive lasagna, sauce and meatballs. All the heavy lifting was done the day before so we could actually enjoy the day with our company. Any animosity I had over Christmas Eve quickly dissipated.

Christmas Day was a smash hit. My entire family showed up. Grown-ups and young-downs alike had a good time. We ate, played games and...wait for it...*sang carols!* Our spiritual harmony manifested in song! Even my father, who had become bellicose over the course of the Trump administration, gave political vitriol a break for the day. The picture of my whole family singing Christmas carols together would now best have been captured by Norman Rockwell instead of Norman Lear! Our family had come a long way, trading anxiety and bitterness for peace and harmony. A true Christmas miracle.

Shortly after the holidays wrapped, we pointed ourselves toward the promise of a new year. I was getting ready for a week-long trip to Puerto Rico with a friend. This Caribbean enclave was on my target list for potential retirement locales. Jim couldn't get the time off work, so we agreed to take another scouting trip together in March. A few days before I left, Jim mentioned that he had a pain in his chest. Upon further discussion, he narrowed it down to the ribs on his left side. He didn't make a big deal about it, so I didn't pay much attention to this new discomfort. Besides, I was preoccupied with getting ready to leave. Upon my return, I was going to be immersed in the work of launching my new executive coaching business. As usual, I had multiple to-do lists running through my head like ticker tape.

Jim wasn't one to visit the doctor for unexplained ailments or pains. In typical fashion, he self-diagnosed. "Maybe I pulled a muscle while lifting weights," he speculated. There had been a similar scenario about 20 years ago. He'd complained of a pain in his chest one morning before I went to work. I was then a personal trainer, and my first client was at five a.m. I brought up Jim's chest pain to my last client of the day as a way to make small talk to keep her mind off her exercise-induced discomfort. Her response scared the bejesus out of me. She told me a story about a young, healthy man who had a "widow maker" heart attack after ignoring a pain in his chest. She was from Texas. Somehow her accent added emphasis to the urgency of her story:

> "He was a young guy! Maybe about 40. And in great shape. I'm tellin' you he just came back from a run. He went into his living room, sat down and that was it. Dead as a door nail. Without any warning. You need to go home right now and get your husband to the hospital!"

Her recounting of this poor guy's untimely demise put me in a flat-out panic. I ran home and insisted Jim go to his doctor. It turned out to be a pulled muscle after all. He was very annoyed with my Chicken Little impression.

Fast forward 20 years, where that relic of an incident did not help my case to get him to seek medical attention for this chest pain. Alas, memories of past wrongs accumulated over time contribute to the mountain of grievances shared by a couple. But I didn't insist or nag him about it. It's not that I worried less 20 years later. Relationships evolve so much over time. One of the things I decided after I turned 50 was that nagging Jim about certain marital "stuck points" like his DIY approach to his own health didn't add any value to our couple-hood, so I stopped. *Jim can take care of his own body and make his own decisions,* I told myself. If there were adverse effects from his decisions, then we'd just have to deal with the consequences as they came. Besides, if I inquired about his plans to mitigate whatever ailed him, it was received as a provocation, not an expression of concern. Engaging him in useless bickering about it wouldn't motivate him to go to the doctor, so why bother? It would only aggravate us both. I didn't pursue the issue and I went to Puerto Rico.

Oddly, during that same week before I left, Jim started asking me about updating our wills. We hadn't updated them in at least 20 years. He became increasingly persistent about tending to this task. Perhaps the pain was bothering him more than he was willing to admit? Did he know subconsciously that something was wrong with his body? I didn't make the connection at the time. His persistence on the subject was uncharacteristic, and I responded with annoyance rather than concern. We split household administrative duties, and retirement funds and wills fell in my category. If Jim had an idea or wanted to have input in my category, he'd harangue me until I addressed the matter. And I did the same to him. We were equal opportunity pains in the ass. This time, I was super annoyed because it seemed he wanted me to deal with it in the three days before I left, and that just wasn't going to happen. Finally, I said to him in exasperation: "What is the big deal? I don't plan on dying in Puerto Rico! We can take care of it when I get back!"

While I was away, I was plagued by an eerie feeling that I couldn't shake. I chalked it up to being in an unfamiliar setting, though I'd never had this feeling in the other places I've traveled. What compounded the weird feeling was that I didn't hear from Jim very much during the week. He'd wait a day or two to respond to my texts. That wasn't cause for alarm, but it felt peculiar. I excused the irregularity in my mind by chalking it up to his busy schedule. When I did hear from him, he sounded preoccupied.

My friend's sister joined our Puerto Rico travel party. Her marriage had a 23-year lead on mine. Her husband had some health problems that she was concerned about as well. It seemed she had done a lot more work on accepting what she could not control than I had. Yes, I decided not to nag my husband about his health, but it still bugged me. I was working on trying to find a way to let it go. I remember expressing my exasperation. I shared with her that I understood this was a psychologically mature approach, but I still thought Jim's behavior was completely unfair. It upset me that if something happened to him as a result of his lack of self-care, I would be the one who had to endure watching him suffer. And, if it was grave? I'd be the one left to pick up the pieces. It's chilling to realize how prescient that conversation was.

That conversation highlighted the conundrum that affects every kind of human relationship. Couples, siblings, parents and friends all grapple with the frustration that results from wanting to control their loved ones' actions. I mean, try asking your 85-year-old father to surrender the keys to his car or getting your young adult daughter to go to the doctor when you're certain she has strep throat. We tell ourselves time and again: "You've got to let people do what they're going to do. You can't control anything but your own actions and responses to the world around you." But damn, working that out is one of the most vexing aspects of interpersonal relationships.

We landed in Rochester at about one a.m., Sunday, January 19th. Jim came to pick me up at the airport as he always did. No matter what time of day or night, Jim insisted on dropping me off and picking me up. For years I traveled around the northeast, often having to be up and out as early as four-thirty. It didn't matter to Jim. He faithfully taxied me to see me off and greet me back home. What makes this seemingly benign activity remarkable is the fact that Jim was decidedly, genetically, unarguably *not* a morning person. Remember the earlier detailed morning scramble he engaged in before work? He was always running late because he had an enviable love affair with sleep. Over the years, I've seen my husband fall asleep mid-sentence while talking to dinner guests. He fell asleep at the wheel once and flipped his truck. He even fell asleep on a treadmill. So, you see, waking from his precious slumber and leaving behind his warm bed to retrieve me from the airport was an incredible act of selflessness that left me feeling loved and cared for.

When he got out of the car to help me with my bags, I was alarmed by his appearance. His complexion was gray, he looked like he hadn't slept in days and he had a persistent cough. He said he had a chest cold. Based on my visual assessment of his symptoms, that sounded about right to me. He told me he went for his regular run on Friday, but had to cut it short because he didn't have the energy to finish. We went right to sleep when we got home but he got up early that Sunday to go help some friends move furniture. (That's the kind of guy Jim was. He was always ready and able to help a friend. Though he wasn't feeling well, he wasn't about to let them down.) When he came home from the moving excursion, he was wiped out. He lay down on the couch and slept for the rest of the day. That night, he couldn't sleep because his original chest pain started radiating to his upper middle back.

Finally, first thing in the morning, he relented. I took him to see his primary care physician. The doctor was on vacation, leaving the physician assistant in charge. She said his left lung didn't sound like it was filling all the way and instructed us to go to the emergency room so Jim's chest could be screened for a potential pulmonary embolism. I gave an "I told you so" look to my husband, not really understanding what a "pulmonary embolism" was.

Little clues along the way hinted at the dire nature of Jim's condition, but I didn't recognize them at the time. The physician assistant for example gave off an incongruous vibe. Though she was sending us to the emergency room, she didn't seem alarmed. It was odd. So, I naively thought, *Okay. Jim is 56. He is fit and active, but he also eats meat and cheese with wild abandon. It would make sense that he was having some type of cardiopulmonary something-or-other. Those are relatively common conditions that can be fixed.*

Do you want to know what's super fun about being the surviving spouse? I don't just replay in my head all the things I think I did wrong while Jim was sick. No, I go ahead and replay all the things I think I did wrong throughout our entire relationship. From the age of 22 right on through to 52. It's this self-guided spelunking tour into the deepest recesses of my mind where I get to visit self-hatred, anger, guilt and shame. I can't control the exaggerated memories that get screened in the movie theater of my mind. My psyche bought a ticket to the worst chamber of horrors it could find. The tour begins with: *Should I have pressed him to go to the doctor sooner?* and *I went to Puerto Rico while cancer was spreading through his body!* and proceed to: *Why didn't I let him stop at the dinosaur museum in Wyoming?! What is wrong with me?!* This spins out of control, until I'm swimming in this mucky swamp populated by memories of selfishness and self-centered behavior. All the mean things I've ever said or did emerge around me like toxic algae blooms. I have 30 years of data from our relationship together. This exercise in self-flagellation is fucking brutal. But the worst part is my emergence from the swamp. The pain is crippling. I gasp for air and let out a full-throated cry that shakes my entire body. "Why?! Why aren't you here? You should be here, telling me 'It's okay.' Or you'll say 'All of that was over years ago. Why are you still dwelling on it? I love you honey. That's all that matters. Non preoccuparti. Ti amo.'"

The awareness that Jim can't be here to hash this or anything else out with me sits on my chest like an anvil. And I can't breathe! I'd give anything for a good argument with Jim, to be followed by the grace of forgiveness and the most amazing hug you could ever imagine. When we hugged, it felt like we shared one heart. We were good at arguing, and we were equally good at making up. That's the point, isn't it? You aren't born knowing the right way to be. You have to learn. Jim and I were little more than kids when we met. We grew up learning how to be a couple while simultaneously learning how to be humans in this world. We made all the mistakes there were to make and logged a bunch of regrets. The stuck points we had were shared along with the countless beautiful moments we created. We always woke up together. Ready for another day of trying to be better.

All this grappling with the messiness of our relationship doesn't end at the edges of our marriage. It extends to our children, to our families, and to our friends. We're all flawed humans trying to work it out. Trading in the warts on my soul for some notion of purity wouldn't be right, because I would have never learned anything. I wouldn't have been prepared to handle adversity. Jim and I would have never grown into the strong couple we became. Weathering the rough and tumble aspects of our relationship prepared us for the most difficult test of our lives. The truth that matters is this: We marched through an apocalypse, chins up, hand in loving hand, and together, we gave that cancer hell.

There's a line in one of the songs from Dr. Seuss's *How the Grinch Stole Christmas* that goes: "Christmas Day will always be, just so long as we have we." From my perspective, the sentiment extends much further than Christmas. It applies to Veterans Day, "Talk Like A Pirate Day," Garbage Day, and Tuesday. As we ride the wild roller coaster of life, the great gift we're given at birth that makes the good times joyful and the bad times bearable, is each other. Every day will always be, just so long as we have we.

CHAPTER TWO

The Emergency Room

We left the doctor's office, went straight to the hospital, and checked into the emergency room with our instructions from the physician assistant. The intake team checked Jim's blood pressure, asked him some questions, and directed him to sit in the waiting room where we festered for seven hours. Throughout the course of the day, I periodically checked at the information desk to find out if Jim would be seen soon. "We'll call you when it's his turn," was the rote response. I called Jim's doctor's office and asked them to please call the Emergency Department to get him in faster. They said they couldn't do anything. They explained they had no influence over the hospital's emergency room. I asked if they would have Jim's doctor call and make a request, as a professional courtesy, to open space for Jim. "Doctor R is on vacation." "I know that, but would you please call him anyways?! If you really think Jim is having some kind of pulmonary event, why wouldn't someone from your office call the ER doctors and express the urgency here?" Whoever I was talking to was exasperated by my persistence. She said she'd call the doctor and relay my urgent message. I'm sure she said that to get me off the phone, because no one from the doctor's office ever called the ER. I was worried, but told myself that if Jim's condition was urgent, the emergency room would make him a priority, and someone from Jim's doctor's office would have called.

Luck was not with us. We walked into the ER on January 20, 2020. It was Martin Luther King, Jr. Day, a vacation day for many. It also happened to be the first sunny, warmish day in a while, and we were in the middle of one of the worst flu seasons on record. All the folks who didn't want to venture out in the snow and yuck over the weekend for their "emergencies" showed up in the ER that day. People were packed like sardines in the waiting room and down the hallways. It was standing room only. If you squinted, you could mistake the place for Calcutta.

Some homeless-looking dude made himself comfortable smack dab in the middle of the cluster, taking up a much-needed patient chair for his respite. Apparently, he was a regular because the hospital staff knew him by name. No emergent ailment brought him to this chaos party. He was just hanging out, enjoying a place to chill. Which might have been fine on any other day, but not when the waiting room was this crowded. A guard came and politely, yet firmly invited him to leave. When he got up, everyone around him recoiled in disgust. I couldn't see anything from my vantage point, and I certainly wasn't going to investigate, but judging from the continuous gagging coming from his chair neighbors, I believe he relieved himself while enjoying the comfort of his seat. A custodian showed up to assess the situation and extend a knowing sympathy to the people around the soiled chair. He announced that he'd be right back with cleaning supplies post haste. Part of that sentence was true. He did come back, but it was an hour later and he didn't bring any cleaning supplies. He hung out at the information desk and chatted with staff like it was coffee break. Several people sitting around the soiled chair complained multiple times to no avail. A woman who had the misfortune of sitting right next to the human HazMat spill struggled to keep from hurling over the nasty that guy left behind, but there was nowhere else for her to be while she waited for her turn.

We continued to listen for Jim's name while other people were called one by one. This is how the call back process went: A staff person would emerge from the door right next to where we were sitting and bellow a name across the sea of people. If the *bellowee* didn't respond, the *bellower* would yell their name a few more times. If that didn't garner a response, the staff person would come back 10 minutes later and call out again. If the sufferer of an alleged emergency still didn't reply, they would get paged over the intercom in case they were on the premises but not in the actual germ pool of a waiting room. I recognize that this scenario may not come as a surprise to many, but for me, a person who has only ever been in an ER twice before, the whole process struck me as oddly inefficient and counterintuitive to helping people in crisis.

At twelve-thirty p.m. I told Jim I was going to run to the grocery store and that he should call me when he was called. I thought for sure he'd be called in by the time I got back. There wasn't any food in the house since I'd been on vacation, and I figured I'd get a quick shop in so we could have dinner when we got home. Though tentative, my brain remained on a normalcy track. None of these health professionals had a sense of urgency where Jim was concerned, so my assumptions about a manageable health situation continued to be reinforced. I called him while I was gone, to check in. He was still in the waiting room. I returned an hour later, fully expecting to find him in a room being assessed by someone. Nope. He was still in the waiting room, looking and feeling worse.

At four o'clock, I went to the desk *again* and asked if Jim was going to be seen. They said they were getting a room ready for him as we spoke. Finally! But another hour went by. At five, a petite Asian woman came out and called Jim's name. We got up and followed her through the door and down the hall. While we were walking with her, she mumbled in a heavy accent "I called you an hour ago." What!? "No you didn't! We were sitting right next to the door!" we replied. It turned into a "Yes I did," "No you didn't!" exchange. I was already on my last nerve, and from my perspective, this attendant was being antagonistic. Why in the world would she even bother to tell us that she called us an hour ago? To scold us? To cover her ass and make it look like she was doing her job? Finally, I said, "Well if you had called us and we didn't answer, why weren't we paged like everyone else?" To which she replied "Paging not good," whatever the hell that meant.

As this inanity played out, we were shown to Jim's holding cell. The full space looked to be about 15 feet x 10 feet. Medical equipment and gurneys took up most of the floor space. A curtain split the room into two patient areas, creating an illusion of privacy. If the curtain had been a wall, each space would have been nothing but a broom closet. It looked like a set-up for a scene from a Marx Brothers movie. Seriously, I was waiting for Groucho to show up in a white coat with a saw in his hand.

The patient sharing the space was only a couple feet away on the other side of the curtain. His visitor was large and loud, sitting in the one and only chair that could fit in the closet. The lack of real estate forced us to share a physical intimacy. If it wasn't for the curtain, passers-by would have thought we were lovers. Every time she stood up, she knocked the chair into me through the curtain, so I moved to the foot of Jim's gurney to claim a small buffer of personal space. At one point, she got on her cell phone and started speaking as if she didn't have a phone at all and was trying to communicate with someone in Antarctica, adding to the circus-like atmosphere. Our neighboring patient had multiple visitors cycling through in addition to his main person, which was concerning to me. If this patient had so many visitors, how long had they been in the closet? Were we going to be here that long? Plus, adding more people made the loud, cramped space even louder and crampter.

By then, Jim was feeling absolutely horrible and had a terrible headache. I felt so bad for him. All he wanted was a Tylenol. Getting a Tylenol in that ER would have been a miracle akin to raising the dead. This brought back memories of the last time Jim wanted something for a headache in that hospital. It was 1994 and we had recently returned from our honeymoon—a camping trip in Allegany State Park. We borrowed mountain bikes from friends for the trip. We decided to take one last ride through the woods behind our house before we returned the bikes. Jim was not an experienced mountain biker by any stretch, but he had all the elasticity a 30-year-old enjoys accompanied by an adventurous spirit. Local enthusiasts had set up an entire bike course which included a big hill with a decent sized mogul at the bottom. There were some local college students riding the course when we got there. We watched for a while. Then Jim decided he was going to give the course a try. When he started down the hill, I turned my back for a second to talk to one of the students. I knew something bad happened by the look on the kid's face. I whipped around and sure enough Jim was flat on his back at the bottom of the hill with the bike on top of him. We all ran down the hill to find 'Evel Knievel' had knocked himself clean out.

The students called 911 while I gently tried to revive Jim. When he came to, he asked: "Where am I?" *Uh-oh,* I thought.

Me: "We're on Pinnacle Hill."

Jim: "How did I get here?"

I started asking questions on a backward timeline to see how much of his memory he'd lost.

Me: "Do you remember taking the bikes off the porch?"

Jim: "No."

Me: "Do you remember borrowing bikes from John & Bryce?"

Jim: "No."

Me: "Do you remember riding in Allegany?"

Jim: "No."

Hmm. This is bad. I thought. *Now we're really in dangerous territory if the answer to this next question isn't what it should be.*

Me: "Do you remember our wedding?"

"We're married?" he exclaimed with disturbed wonder. "Oh my God!"

I almost hit him in the head to knock everything back in place.

The EMT's showed up and strapped Jim to a backboard. He was transported to this same ER where he waited, immobilized on the backboard, for about five hours. It should come as no surprise that he developed a headache. He asked someone for a Tylenol. A young woman showed up with a syringe filled with Percocet. She didn't tell us who she was and she wasn't wearing a badge with identification. For all we knew, she'd wandered in off the street. As for Jim, he didn't want to be off his tits. He simply wanted a Tylenol for his headache. She didn't hide her extreme irritation when he declined the shot.

Back to our current situation, we asked a person we assumed was a nurse for Tylenol. (Twenty years later and still no credentialling introduction. How comforting to know the absence of identification remained *de rigueur* in their emergency room. At least they're consistent?) She had to ask another person who had to have another person enter the request in the computer for a doctor to authorize the request. Someone else had to follow the order in the computer to see when it was authorized so they could have another person go get the Tylenol and give it to someone to administer it to Jim. This is what the health system has become. As soon as you cross the threshold of a hospital, you leave personhood behind and become a liability to the health professionals and an expense to the insurers. I was kicking myself because I didn't have my purse with me. No self-respecting woman leaves home without pain medication. If I'd remembered it, we could've avoided this nonsense.

While that process was working itself through, someone came in to take blood samples. At about six-thirty p.m., they wheeled Jim back to have a CT scan of his chest. When the imaging was finished, he was parked in a hallway outside the scan room, waiting for someone to return him to the closet. There were still so many people all over the place it looked like a MASH unit. We were in the hallway for about a half an hour when the CT technician emerged from his room and exclaimed: "Oh! No one has come to get you yet?" He chatted with us for a brief bit. He told us the ER was the busiest he'd ever seen it. Then he said: "I'll wheel you back." The guy's friendliness was greatly appreciated. He was the first person who treated us like humans. He parked Jim back in the closet and parted by saying: "Good luck!" That's when I started to suspect something was really wrong. This man had seen the inside of Jim's chest. He was gentle and kind with Jim as mayhem swirled around us. And, he went out of his way to make Jim comfortable, doing someone else's job by bringing him back to the emergency room. All that, tied with a "good luck" bow, gave me pause.

We continued to wait. It was going on seven-thirty when a resident came in to talk to us. He was a handsome young Indian man who looked like he'd seen a ghost. He told us that they looked at Jim's CT scan and blood work. What followed was unexpected, unwanted and shocking news. The resident said they found a mass in Jim's chest. His white blood cell count was abnormally high and his lymph nodes were swollen. The doctors suspected cancer, but they weren't sure what kind. He said that the ER oncology resident would be in shortly to talk to us. While he was trying to deliver this news, our closet neighbor's visitor knocked into him several times while shouting to Antarctica again. He was competing with her volume-wise, while attempting to sensitively and caringly tell Jim he had cancer. The whole thing was chaotic, surreal and inhumane.

We weren't the only ones shocked by this news. That poor kid totally drew the short straw. To this day, I honestly feel bad for him. I think he was a first-year resident, and this may have been the first time he had to deliver terrible news under deplorable conditions.

Though we heard the word "cancer," we didn't yet understand the severity of Jim's illness. All I knew was that my husband looked and felt terrible, we were surrounded by a chamber of horrors, and we had just received terrifying news. At that point, all I wanted to do was go home. The resident scurried off to summon the chief ER doctor in order to prevent an ill-advised exit. Upon her arrival, I told her we wanted to leave. She did her very best not to freak out. In hindsight, I understand why. While Jim's symptoms didn't seem much worse than a chest cold, they were indicative of something critical. She said they *strongly* advised we *not* go home and that a room was being prepared for Jim in the cancer center as we spoke.

What?! This can't be! I thought. None of this was sinking in fast enough. Certainly not as fast as the cancer was spreading through Jim's body. *He's probably the healthiest, most active 56-year-old anyone has ever met.* Now we were being told that our lives were changing drastically and would never be the same because we were entering a horrid, horrid world. My brain was stunned. It was going to take a while for it to catch up to the room. I never wished for a pulmonary embolism so badly.

The oncology resident came in while we were still in the "closet." He was a delicate looking man who spoke softly and confidently. He was kind and measured as he explained that Jim would be admitted into the cancer center of the hospital. He said they suspected Jim had leukemia, and that he would need to undergo a series of tests to verify the diagnosis and determine the actual type of leukemia.

That's when the *What? What? What?* loop started playing in my head.

CHAPTER THREE

Everyone Equals No One

Shortly after our conversation with the oncology resident in the ER, Jim was admitted to the cancer center. After 11 hours with all of our emergency room friends, going to the cancer center was like checking in to a spa. Despite the upgrade, I knew the charm would wear off quickly.

A number of people cycled through the room to talk to us, then hurried off. Though the hyper-activity was fast becoming a blur, I was able to grasp the fact that they needed to start running tests on Jim immediately in order to understand what kind of cancer he had. Finally, after languishing unnoticed in the ER, there was a sense of urgency around Jim's care. It now felt like the doctors were working to get ahead of the sands in the hour glass. The cancer was moving quickly. The sooner they figured out the type of leukemia Jim had, the faster they could create a treatment plan to start beating it back.

The next morning, we were introduced to Jim's dedicated "team." Before I describe this meeting, I'll share that *my* definition of a team is a group of people brought together with complementary strengths and skills to collaborate for the purpose of achieving a common goal. A team has a coach who is ultimately accountable for the team's actions. The coach is adept at creating work environments and processes that are conducive to cooperation and collaboration so the team can hit that sweet spot of efficiency and peak performance. Without a coach, a team is rudderless—it can settle into groupthink, get pushed off course by a dominant player and generally run amok.

The doctors who showed up that morning were proud to introduce us to our dedicated healthcare "team," which seemed to consist of about 100 people, most of whom looked like they were the age of our kids. It quickly became clear that we did not have a shared definition of "team." I guess if one's idea of a team is a group of people standing next to each other, then sure, it was a team. From my vantage point, however, this group of people standing next to each other seemed to be more like a mob.

The introductions felt like a well-choreographed sales pitch. Roswell Park Cancer Center, one of our cancer center's big competitors, is a mere hour away, so I guess they wanted to put their best effort into a "Ta-Da!"-like moment so we wouldn't be tempted to go elsewhere. "We're your team! You can call on us for anything! We're *all* here for *you!* I'm Dr. so and so, this is Dr. so and so, this is nurse so and so," etc. When I started to ask who was a doctor and who was a resident, a sense of discomfort entered the room. Our discomfort was already off the charts, but I guess there's always room for more. There was a lot of weight shifting and shoe scrutiny. I understand that yes, a resident is a doctor. However, I wanted to know who in the room had the years of experience with Jim's disease. It was becoming abundantly clear that Jim's diagnosis was serious. I didn't want to sift through 50 people to get to the expert.

We were in peak crisis mode. Our new healthcare "team" was focused on presenting their flat organizational model to a man who was critically ill, exhausted and in shock. No one person emerged as the coach who was responsible for organizing this crowd of people in our room. This introduction was not well thought out from the patient perspective. If one inquiry had managed to surface from the cacophony of questions clanging in my head, I wouldn't have known where to direct it because I was addressing an audience. An audience, by the way, that didn't display any evidence of genuine human emotion. It was unsettling. While one person talked, the rest of the group stared at us without showing any affect. Jim and I felt like Donald Sutherland and Brooke Adams in *Invasion of the Body Snatchers*. Later, we found that individually, many of these providers were personable. But as a "mob", they were like zombies. Suffice it to say, this presentation did not instill confidence. When they finished with their grand presentation, familiar words came out of my mouth. Words I used to say all the time when I worked in banking: "Everyone equals no one." My words were met with blank stares.

As it turned out, we also did not have a shared definition of the word "dedicated." What was left out of that initial presentation was that our dedicated team was only *dedicated* from 9 a.m. to 5 p.m., Monday through Friday, for a few weeks. Give or take. Then a new team would rotate in. There was a nightly shift change with completely different people who weren't part of our team *per se*, but one of them had a team member's phone number. Weekends were an entirely different story. There were a lot less people and they were not our team either. They were people who kept the ball rolling until Monday morning. And of course, team members get sick and have vacation time, so odds are you won't see the team you met on day one in its original configuration ever again. It's best not to have any major issues at night, on the weekends or during the holidays. In addition, there are more teams from other departments who will rotate through to check other presenting issues who have nothing to do with the original team. No one from your team accompanies those departmental teams, so you won't have any feeling of continuity or confidence that any one person has the whole picture in mind and is really looking out for you.

The team members took turns talking at a brisk tempo in controlled, monotone voices. It felt like someone was throwing small rocks at my head in rapid succession while my arms were pinned to my sides. The last person to talk ended their dissertation with what came across as feigned empathy: "I know it's a lot. Do you have any questions?" Huh, let me see. We are standing here, paralyzed with fear and drenched by a fire hose of information. What should my question be? Can I buy a fucking vowel? My brain was sparking like an old toaster about to catch fire while it tried to process all of this information. As I stood there, mouth agape and eyes glazed, everyone left the room, mistaking my paralysis for: "No questions? Ok, well you can call us any time if you do have questions." Yeah, right. By the time I could talk, the entire team had rotated out. Even the social worker, who might be an appropriate person to provide some continuity, gave a rapid 10-minute info dump after the "team" left, before scurrying off to meet other patient demands. By then, my head felt like a speed bag.

Finding a team member in the first week turned into a treasure hunt. What we ultimately learned was that if you have a question, ask your (current) nurse who will ask or leave a message for someone else. During that process, lots of other things will happen like cancer, pain, sadness, fear, and the demands of our lives outside the hospital. You almost forget what the heck you asked until the impetus for the question recurs, and then you try to track down where your question ended up in the process. Which is likely nowhere because it "slipped through the cracks at shift change" so you start all over again with your new nurse. Everyone equals no one.

In hindsight, I realize that my anger and irritations were ignited by ambiguous processes and systems, rather than by individuals. Holistic health *care* of a person is greatly diminished when one enters a health *system*. It's not crazy talk to say that supporting a holistic approach to the health *care* of an individual is more likely to achieve improved health outcomes as opposed to viewing someone in pieces. Throughout the week, Jim felt more and more like the scarecrow from the Wizard of Oz after the flying monkeys tossed his body parts all over the place.

> *"They tore my legs off and they threw them over there. Then they tore my chest out and they threw it over there!"*

We were desperately clinging to every piece of information and trying to organize it in a way that made sense to us. Our struggling minds wanted to buy into the team concept because it created an expectation of care continuity. But the constant revolving door of people, places and equipment did not align with that concept. It's no exaggeration to say that you could fill a lecture hall with all of the people who saw Jim in that first week. The mismanagement of our expectations was cruel.

What we really needed was one person who could help guide our education on Jim's disease, explain the complexity of care options and the resulting effects, connect us to a wider breadth of relevant patient information and resources and give the "heads up" on what we could expect with each step. All I remember receiving in that first week was a piece of paper that said his cancer had a 90% remission rate. I later learned that those statistics didn't apply to someone Jim's age.

It seemed like everyone we talked to had a paper and pencil set when we needed the person with the Crayola 120 pack, complete with crayon sharpener. Hell, I would have settled for someone with the 64 pack. I've since learned that some cancer centers have professionals on staff called "patient navigators." This person has all the crayons. The absence of such a guiding hand on our team left us feeling lost and alone under a cloudy sky much of the time. A dull gray outlook doesn't inspire hope.

CHAPTER FOUR

From Worse to Worser

Throughout the course of our second day in the hospital, Jim underwent a series of tests and scans before he was prepped for a bone marrow biopsy. Though all those other tests were necessary health status indicators, the pathology from the biopsy would inform the doctors as to the exact type of leukemia he had. I didn't know there were so many.

The biopsy procedure involved the insertion of a metal straw into the back of Jim's hip bone so they could extract some of his bone marrow. They told us that these rapidly multiplying cancer cells make a person's bones more dense, therefore more difficult to puncture with a metal straw. Our natural assumption was that Jim would be sedated for the procedure because getting pierced in your bone sounds fucking painful.

For some bizarre reason, this reminds me of Jim's vasectomy. Jim and I knew after our second son was born, a short 18 months after our first, that our capacity for parenthood was maxed. I'm not going to go so far as to say that we were good at man-to-man defense but we at least felt like we had a fighting chance. If we had ventured into zone defense by bringing in a third Baby Barbero, our spirits could've been crushed and our children might well have ended up as feral cretins roaming the streets.

The sterilization conversation usually came up in the middle of the night while we were being serenaded by wailing babies. *"You do it!" "No, you do it!"* we would shout over the shrieks of our progeny. Our inability to agree on who was going to get "procedured" was a significant speed bump on our road to terminating our procreating abilities.

The one thing that worked to my advantage was Jim's thrift. Initially, this compounded the problem because our health insurance didn't cover the procedure for either of us. But like a message from God, who was probably taking pity on us because we hadn't slept in a year, a quarter page ad for a free vasectomy appeared in our community paper. *Ha! Problem solved!* I thought. I eagerly showed the ad to Jim. Well, 'free vasectomy' didn't quite ignite his enthusiasm like it did mine. But I was not going to let this opportunity escape. In the next few weeks, the ad kept appearing, but the doctors advertising started charging a nominal fee that increased with each week. When it hit $20, I knew my window was closing. We both did our share of investigating to make sure this wasn't a weird science experiment or that the word "veterinary" wasn't hidden somewhere in the ad. After everything checked out, we made a consultation appointment with the doctor advertising. He told us that they were practicing a non-traditional procedure that involved using a poke hole to get to the vas deferens rather than making an incision. He said many of the men going through the procedure don't need any anesthesia and had much shorter recovery periods than with the traditional method. In fact, he told us many men go right back to work after this type of vasectomy.

I was completely sold. Go ahead! Poke my husband in the nuts! Stop the madness! Jim was lukewarm at best, but the kids weren't getting any quieter and the price was right, so he acquiesced. In hindsight, it's like "Somnolence" was the name of a person living in our house, driving bad decisions early on in our parenting days.

I accompanied Jim to the appointment. There were two men in the waiting room outfitted in construction gear. The first guy was called back. 20 minutes later, he walked out, no worse for the wear. The second guy was called back. He too walked out 20 minutes later as if nothing happened. It appeared the doctor wasn't exaggerating about the easy recovery. Then, it was Jim's turn. I went into the exam room with him. As soon as the doctor touched Jim in his nether region, he started flopping around on the table like a fresh-caught fish on a dock. Unlike a fish, we couldn't hit him on the head with a mallet to get him to sit still. We all tried talking him through it to no avail. He could not let this procedure go through without some kind of sedation. The doctors gave up and pulled out a syringe filled with "night-night" juice. The drug cocktail was a fast acting, short-lived sedation that gave me a small window of time to make a couple inappropriate jokes at my husband's expense while the doctors did their work. When they were done, Jim snapped to and walked out without any issue. Now, we could continue caring for our baby demons with the confidence of people who knew that no new yowls were going to be joining the midnight chorus.

All these years later, nothing about our current situation had any of the levity present during Jim's vasectomy. So imagine our dismay upon learning that this procedure was going to be performed without any sedation. This was not gonna go well. *Where is the vasectomy doctor and his magic syringe?*

Jim was a nervous wreck in anticipation. His body was so tensed up, I imagined they were going to need a jackhammer to get through his muscles before they could touch his hip bone. They numbed the external area and gave him an antianxiety medication in advance with the hope that he would relax, but that did not work. I felt so unprepared. I tried to play music for him through his phone in a lame attempt to distract him—a fiasco on my part. I couldn't figure out his phone or how his streaming service worked. The music I played when I finally figured it all out didn't provide any distraction or comfort whatsoever. All I could do was hold his hand and talk to him softly while they pierced him in the back.

The atmosphere in the room itself was funereal. The metal straw had to cut through the tension in the room before it could even touch Jim's back. The nurse performing the procedure did an amazing job. He got in and out as quickly as possible, extracting what he needed. Though he was nimble and seemingly quick, it still hurt like a mother and I'm sure to Jim it felt like hours were dragging by. Jim and I let out a collective sigh of relief that could be heard on the other side of the hospital when the nurse was done. Now we had to wait while the folks in the lab analyzed the biopsied blood sample.

At the end of this exhausting day, Jim's blood oxygen level started to fall. He'd already lived through a horrible day. All he wanted was a little rest while he processed the cancer news. Clearly rest wasn't on his body's agenda that night. Less than 24 hours after his preliminary diagnosis, an even bigger health emergency was presenting.

Around 11 p.m., all manner of healthcare professionals came piling into his room with a bunch of medical equipment. The new activity conveyed a sense of urgency, but everyone went about their tasks quietly and calmly. Their body language was sending mixed messages, which made it difficult for me to gauge the severity of the situation.

A nurse stuck a needle in Jim's hand, which was a painful surprise judging from the sound of a swallowed yelp coming from Jim. Then they poked and prodded him as more people came in with additional equipment. There was nothing I could do but watch the flurry of activity. I was becoming increasingly agitated because everything they did seemed to hurt Jim and I couldn't connect the activity with a reason or purpose. I kept saying "His blood oxygen level was just at 100%. It's only down slightly. He looks fine. He's not acting any different. What's going on?!" At this point, all I was told was that Jim had to be transported to the Intensive Care Unit (ICU). The physician assistant was doing a poor job of explaining why all the interventions were required. A look of exasperation came across his face that indicated he was losing patience with my inability to decipher what I perceived as his antiseptic tiptoeing around the truth. But there were big gaps in the information being conveyed. It seemed he was afraid of telling me how serious all this was. Despite his frustration, I continued to press him for answers. My voice rose, and with a frantic urgency I squawked: "I can't help but feel that there is something you aren't telling me! Why is all this happening!? Why are we going to the ICU?!" No longer interested in being part of this conversation, he grabbed his assistant and shoved her between us, creating enough of a diversion for him to execute his escape. *Fuck you very much.* I thought as I watched him saunter down the hall. Meanwhile, the stand-in stared at me with an unnerving, frozen smile on her face. To this day, I would give anything to punch him in his face as hard as I could, and slap that look off the resident's mug so she would never smile that vacant smile at anyone ever again.

So, what exactly was happening to Jim? Here are the medical notes from that morning: "Patient found to have a large anterior Mediastinal mass with a white blood cell count of 80, 41% miscellaneous cells (most likely blasts) highly concerning for a high-grade lymphoma. The CT scan also showed bilateral pleural effusions and a pericardial effusion, meeting tamponade physiology. This is a critically ill patient with the potential to decompensate quickly due to tumor lysis syndrome, tamponade physiology and acute hypoxic respiratory failure." That "potential to decompensate quickly" described in the morning notes was realized that night.

Seeing as crises don't typically afford one the opportunity to Google search medical terms, the following explanation would have been much more useful to me: "Jennifer, your husband is in danger of going into heart failure because the cancer cells are multiplying so quickly, his blood is turning into sludge." *That* I would have understood. But it was after hours so our "dedicated team" wasn't there. I had the night shift, who all seemed to be crabby and they either didn't think it was important for me to understand what was happening, or they were afraid to tell me just how critical Jim was. It turns out that this crabby group of people was the rapid response team. They swarm in when a patient is in critical condition. No one told me that's who they were. I found out from reading Jim's medical records one year later.

During this round of chaos, they outfitted Jim with a BiPap machine that looked like a clear Darth Vader helmet. You could see Jim's face, but you couldn't hear him very well. His voice was dull and echoey inside the helmet, competing with the loud rushing sound of oxygen being pumped in. Around two a.m. they wheeled him to the medical intensive care unit on the other side of the hospital.

The cancer center nurses instructed me to remove all our things from the room. I had to take our stuff back to my car like a wandering nomad in the middle of the night. Then, I had to find my way through the labyrinthine hospital corridors to where Jim was being held in intensive care. Once there, I sat next to him, watching all the monitors as intensely as one would watch a psychological thriller. Though it was late, sleep was elusive because I was so wired from the freneticism of the last 48 hours.

To help you better understand my state of mind during this medical pandemonium, I'm going to share a few of my previous hospital experiences. Experiences that have rendered me intensely afraid of being a patient in a hospital. *Especially* a teaching hospital. It doesn't mean that I don't appreciate the education necessary to train the future generations of doctors and nurses. I'm sure I've benefited from the medical science learned in these teaching settings and for that I'm grateful. It's very easy for me to be appreciative when I'm not in the hospital. But if it's me or my loved ones, appreciation quickly gets crowded out by fear and hatred.

I suppose it goes back to the birth of our younger son Gianni. Early in the morning the day after he was born, bruising appeared on his abdomen and one of his testicles looked like a purple globe grape. I hadn't seen the bruising yet because we were still resting. Less than 24 hours prior, I had given birth, without pain medication, to an almost 10-pound baby. And no, I was not against pain meds. The little guy was in a hurry to come out, so there wasn't enough time for the anesthesia people to numb me up before pushing a bowling ball out of my vagina. It's no exaggeration on my part to say that I resembled the many women TV shows and comedians have satirized for years because I literally shrieked: "This is a hospital! There's gotta be something you can give me!" When the nurse examined Gianni, she found the bruising and freaked out. An appropriate reaction I'd say. She called another nurse in for a second set of professional eyes on the situation. That person immediately assumed an accusatory posture with Jim. We didn't get what they were implying because it never occurred to us that child abuse was a possibility. Looking back, I'm sadly aware that they'd seen terrible things. And yet, at the risk of sounding jaded, I also figure their ego defenses told them that if Jim was to blame, they weren't.

The nurses summoned the resident to look at Gianni. After a brief examination, she looked me straight in the eyes and said they would have to remove his testicle because it hadn't dropped properly and it was too late to save it. I was dumbfounded. Though I was unable to speak, the look of horror on my face communicated plenty. The nurse standing behind her decided to add to the excitement by chiming in with: "You're just upset because of postpartum hormones." It's a good thing she was out of my reach. My fist wanted to give her an up-close look at the effects of "postpartum hormones."

They ran a bunch of tests on Gianni, including X-rays and ultrasounds. My pediatrician was out of town so I didn't have anyone I could trust to help us navigate this insanity. That evening the chief resident marched into my room, noticeably pissed. He was a tall man who walked with an air of authority. I was sitting in an easy chair nursing Gianni when he started asking me questions in a brusque, staccato manner. He asked me if the baby was eating ok. I replied: "Yes."

Dr.: "Is your baby pooping?"

Me: "Yes."

Dr.: "Is he sleeping?"

Me: "Yes."

Dr.: "Does your baby seem okay to you?"

Me: "Yes."

He then stood bolt upright, looked at the wall above my head and announced in an angry tone to what seemed to be an imaginary audience: "There is nothing wrong with this baby!" Then he spun around on his heel and marched out. Thank God for that guy. That's the last I heard of anyone cutting off my son's testicle.

That alone should have been enough to turn me off of teaching hospitals. But there were other incidents that friends and I experienced over the years—my subconscious took notes and organized them in the emergency files of my mind. I noticed for example that when I had minor procedures, the doctors wouldn't tell me straight up that a resident was performing them. I found out that this was common through a physician friend. That lack of transparency was pretty dodgy and certainly did not engender trust.

Another frightening situation happened to the wonderful minister who officiated at our kids' baptisms. Sadly, she became sick with some weird autoimmune disease. When I went to visit her in the hospital one day, she was very upset. A doctor had taken her in for an unscheduled surgery a few nights prior. Myriad complications cascaded after this late-night procedure. She thought being operated on at night was suspect and warned me very seriously from her hospital bed: "Don't ever let anyone operate on you in the middle of the night!" She felt like she had been experimented on.

All this information over time got tucked away in my brain, to be recalled in the early days of Jim's care. When all those people showed up in Jim's room in the middle of the night the second day we were in the hospital, I think it's understandable why I just about lost my shit. And the lack of clear communication was an extra straw too many.

We woke the next morning to an atmosphere imbued with high energy. The cancer center is much more chill by comparison. The ICU rooms were smaller, with many more patients in close proximity. Not as bad as the ER. I mean shit—nothing is as bad as that ER. But there was definitely a greater sense of urgency in the air. There were as many flashing lights as an airport and all kinds of beeps and buzzes could be heard up and down the hallways. Despite the situational stress of intensive care, the doctor in charge was calm, and genuinely kind. After Jim had been handed off to so many different people in such a short period of time, I was pleasantly surprised by the fact that we got to see this doctor fairly regularly. The consistency was comforting.

It was here in the ICU where I found out that our dedicated team wasn't our team anymore for two reasons. First, we had moved to the other side of the hospital. Though Jim was a cancer patient, he was no longer considered a patient of the cancer center. Essentially, we had entered Walmart in the lawn and garden section, and in the middle of the night they moved us to the grocery section. Much like Walmart, if you ask someone in one department about a product from another department, you might as well have asked them about the cost of real estate in the City of Atlantis.

Second, Jim had entered the hospital in the third week of a three-week rotation. That meant all the doctors and residents we met during our initial team orientation were in the process of tapping out. The attending from our first team did end up visiting us, but we were never sure when she was going to show up. If I was in the bathroom or the cafeteria, I missed my chance to talk to her. Waiting for the doctors was a common theme throughout our entire hospital experience. My corporate brain was accustomed to strict schedules that were filled with meetings taking place at times mutually agreed upon by all parties. That's not how it worked here. We learned quickly that the healthcare process culture we were in the midst of was distressingly willy-nilly. Even the best Lean Six Sigma nerds would walk out of here and directly into a bar after five minutes.

Jim was tethered to multiple monitors and machines. There were tubes, cords and wires all over the place. Jim was uncomfortable and the whole scene was disconcerting. He looked like a grounded parade balloon. Just when I thought they couldn't possibly attach anything else, two cancer center nurses came in to insert a Peripherally Inserted Central Catheter, or PICC line for short, into his arm. This would be the access point by which the chemo and other medicines would be administered directly into Jim's veins. A PICC line avoids having to poke a patient repeatedly. The lines looked like funky Christmas tree ornaments dangling from his arm. While they were inserting the line, one of the nurses told me about the importance of properly sterilizing the connection ends. He was very specific as he looked directly at me and said, "These lines need to be sterilized with an alcohol wipe for 20 seconds before and after use. Do NOT let anyone skip this step. An infection can be delivered directly into his system from this line if it isn't sterilized properly." I got the message loud and clear. Turns out, non-cancer-center nurses did not get that memo. I argued with more nurses in the ICU about the sterilization process than you could want to imagine. I had to make them call the cancer center for verification and put a note in Jim's chart, yet the attention to the oncology department's sterilization process remained inconsistent until we got back to the cancer center. One wonders who kept track of this important detail for patients who don't have anyone with them.

Jim's long hair started to get tangled up in all the machine wires and cords. Hair loss was not in Jim's genes, so shortly after he turned 50, he started to grow it out into one fantastically long, lush head of hair. I'm not sure what inspired him to grow it, but I'm glad he did. Maybe it was a middle-aged man's testament to virility? A "screw you" to aging? I don't know. But the long hair added quite nicely to his Samson-like masculine aura.

Acting as an unintentional Delilah, I summoned our trusted family hair manager, Jill. She apparated before our eyes with a bag of salon accoutrements. (Stylists are a special breed. They'd rather be attacked by killer bees than let their clients walk around looking busted.) The boys had joined us in the room. Together we discussed what style Jim should go with. We all settled on a Keanu Reeves à la John Wick. When Jill was finished, Jim's hair fell satisfyingly past his ears, but it was shaped in a way that helped keep it from getting caught in the medical equipment. Now that he had a hospital-friendly haircut, he decided to grow his facial hair. Keep it all simple so he didn't have to fuss with shaving, I guess. Pre-cancer, I never liked a beard on Jim because it was like kissing a wire brush. He only shaved on my account. Now, he was going to go full guns with beard and mustache. He had lost control over his life literally overnight. I certainly wasn't going to protest his defiant middle finger to forces beyond his control.

His connection to machines, tubes and all else rendered him unable to shower, so the nurses gave me packages of warm wet naps and no-rinse shampoo shower caps designed specifically for this purpose. The modern-day sponge bath. Helping him with his ablutions in this weird setting was simultaneously sad and tender.

Over the next couple of days, the critical nature of Jim's health status gradually de-escalated. He was back to his good nature, chatting with the nurses and walking laps around the hospital floor. Though Jim seemed to be feeling better, we were still in limbo, waiting for the results of the tests that would reveal the exact category of his disease.

CHAPTER FIVE

Violated

Late in the afternoon on the fourth day of our hospital stay, we met Jim's oncologist. Finally, a lighthouse in the storm. Doctor B came into Jim's room with one other doctor—an oncology fellow—rather than the crowd we'd come to expect. Though I appreciated the scaled-back approach, in hindsight I realize that for the conversation we were about to have, the professional she should have had with her was a therapist, not a young doctor in training.

The oncologist was unhurried in her explanation of Jim's leukemia, taking great care to make sure we understood his cancer. She explained that after thorough testing, they were able to determine that Jim had something called T-cell acute lymphoblastic leukemia, or T-cell ALL. She actually drew a picture of it to help us visualize the disease.

We learned that leukemia is not as prevalent as other cancers such as breast and lung. For example, in the United States, roughly 60,000 new cases of leukemia are diagnosed a year, compared to 280,000 new cases of breast cancer and 250,000 new cases of lung cancer.

The types of leukemia are grouped into four categories:
- Acute myeloid (or myelogenous) leukemia (AML)
- Chronic myeloid (or myelogenous) leukemia (CML)
- Chronic lymphocytic leukemia (CLL)
- Acute lymphoblastic leukemia (ALL)

About 9.5% of leukemias fall into the ALL category. Annually in the United States, 40% of ALL diagnoses are in adults and 25% of the adult ALL diagnoses are T-cell. That translates into roughly a mere 600 new adult T-cell ALL diagnoses in the U.S. each year. In other words, Jim won Hell's lottery.

Dr. B told us that Jim's disease was progressing rapidly. She said that the steroid he'd been given was a temporary fix, and that chemotherapy was the treatment necessary to give us a shot at driving the cancer into remission. After telling us what the chemotherapy entailed, she said it was her recommendation that Jim begin treatments right away. Sadly, there weren't any other treatment options. There *was* the option of doing nothing, but that most certainly meant death in the near term.

Even if we wanted a second opinion, this aggressive, rapidly moving disease didn't allow for the mind space one would prefer when faced with a life and death decision. We had to place all our trust in Dr. B. There was nothing Jim and I knew that could be of any use in this situation. We had nowhere else to turn. She was *the one.* Our team's coach.

Dr. B further explained that if they could get Jim's cancer in remission, a bone marrow transplant would be their recommended course of action to prevent the mutated cells from coming back. Essentially, they had to kill the malignancy in his bone marrow before they could attempt to give Jim a cellular rebirth. If we agreed to the recommended course of action, she would start him on a chemotherapy regimen that evening. They would proceed with his treatments based on how Jim's body responded to the therapy. Before we could proceed, they needed Jim to sign a consent form. We were terrified and in shock. We don't know how long Jim would've lived if he'd decided to forgo treatment, but judging from his situation in the ICU, I don't think it would have been very long.

What exactly is this aggressive intruder that turned our lives upside down in an instant? Here's my "Dick and Jane" description of T-cell ALL: Different types of blood cells are made in your bone marrow. One type is a white blood cell called a T-cell. These buggers fight off infection. This particular disease affects those infection fighters. But these wily cancer cells are clever survivors, disguising themselves so that other infection fighting cells don't recognize the cancerous T-cells for the imposters they are.

It's like if Wonder Woman, Batman, Superman and all the other superheroes in the Justice League lost their superpowers and turned to a life of crime while maintaining their superhero appearances. The police would be like "Hey, check out Superman helping that old lady into the bank! What a great dude!" Meanwhile, Superman is actually going into the bank to steal from the old lady and everyone else so he can feed his meth habit.

Then, the fallen superheroes start multiplying rapidly. But the replicants are all underdeveloped mutants that have no infection fighting abilities. Their only superpower is exponential reproduction. The mutated superheroes are all spazzy, like 16-year-olds going to a party at a friend's house whose parents are away. As they gather at the party, they collect in and around the pool. They continue to multiply, crowding out everything in the yard. The landscaping gets trompled, and the shed with all the yard tools is crushed. Eventually, the multitudes displace all the water in the pool.

This pool party of mutated T-cells was taking place in Jim's thymus, an important central lymph node, creating a mass in his mediastinum. The mediastinum is the area of the chest that separates the lungs. It's surrounded by the breastbone in front, the spine in back, and the lungs on each side. It contains the heart, aorta, esophagus, thymus, trachea, lymph nodes and nerves. Essentially, most of the important-for-living body parts. It's a terrible place for a rave.

To temporarily corral these superhero-turned-teenage-criminal-ravers, the emergency responders had to hit them with a steroid stun gun. This would keep them at bay until the SWAT team arrived with a Ghostbuster proton pack filled with chemotherapy—cancer's Kryptonite.

The tiny window we had to make a treatment decision further elevated our stress levels. There was no time to sleep on it. Jim had already hit a critical point in the progression of the disease. The partygoers would be up again soon, emboldened in their effort to wreak havoc.

Giving consent is as much a "no" as it is a "yes."

"No, I don't want to die."

"Yes, you can poison me."

Cancer patients are forced into an appalling double bind. *Consent to treatment* is legalese for: "I willingly accept an invitation to be brutally tortured for an indefinite amount of time with the hope that one day I will get to live cancer-free." I vaguely remember Dr. B talking about the risks and side effects that might accompany treatment, but that seemed a mere footnote in my mind compared to the "How do we make this go away?" part of the discussion.

Though Dr. B took her time explaining the disease to us, she did so without knowing anything about our values and life priorities. How could she, or any other person for that matter who just met us? In 30 minutes, 20 of which were dedicated to a didactic lecture on leukemia, how could anyone learn about your character, morals, goals, and aspirations? How could you know if we were religious or nihilists? If we preferred quality of life over quantity? How could you know what someone's humanistic priorities are outside of 'live or die?' Absent that knowledge, how does any doctor know what level of emphasis to place on the 'risks and side effects' part of the discussion? How do they know if it should be the denominator or the numerator in the decision-making calculus?

I have the impression that doctors present information to patients using a combination of science and professional judgment. When you think about it, that's an exceptionally powerful yet precarious position to be in. Inclusion education teaches us that when we don't have time to think something through, unconscious bias grabs the steering wheel of our judgment. We'd all like to think that highly educated medical minds are able to embrace mindfulness as they process the information they have to deliver to a patient. But healthcare professionals are being stretched to perform increasingly more tasks in shorter amounts of time. These conditions are both antithetical *and* antagonistic to mindfulness.

When Giacomo was one year old, we discovered that he had high levels of lead in his blood. It was June of 1999 and Jim was deeply engaged in what became an every-other-year event: painting our house. The troubling news of Giacomo's out-of-whack blood chemistry surfaced in the midst of Jim's fervor. At the young age of 35, Jim approached his inaugural house painting task with vim and vigor. He set his sights on tackling the whole megillah by himself; a two-story, 2,000 square foot home with three different porches. This was a formidable yet doable job for one young man.

This particular summer I was profoundly annoyed because it was hotter than hell and I was four months pregnant with Gianni. Four months pregnant you say? What's the big deal? My pregnancy with Gianni was much different than my first. With Giacomo I didn't show until late in the second trimester. And then, I had a cute little basketball of a pregnant belly. Gianni was a completely different story. I looked and felt like I was 14 months pregnant from the point of conception. Seriously, I was the size of a whale. I literally felt the urge to emit whale sounds every time I had to get up from a chair.

We didn't have central air or any air conditioning window units. In our early life together, Jim's fear of money scarcity bordered on phobic. He wouldn't buy an air conditioner for our room and told me to sit in front of a fan. This was one of those times when I seriously questioned my choice of spouse.

One day Giacomo toddled out onto the porch and bit the wood railing. As I was swiping the chunk of porch out of his mouth I thought, *Huh. I wonder if there's lead in this paint?* I went out back and called up to Jim who was on the ladder, shirtless and in cut-off shorts—the outfit he wore when he did most of his summertime construction projects. "Hey hun? Is there lead in this paint?" To which he replied while scraping away without any tarps, masks or appropriate health and safety equipment: "Probably. The house was built in 1920. I think they stopped using lead in 1945." *Crap.* I chiseled a paint chip from the porch and sent it to the county health department.

The county workers called me two days later and urged me to take Giacomo for a blood test as soon as possible. Sure enough, he had a high blood lead level. It wasn't high enough for him to be chelated, but it definitely clanged the alarm bell at the health department. So much so that government officials swarmed our home like bees. I'm not making this up when I tell you that once we got everything under control, we became the local spokes-family for childhood lead testing.

About a month before that fresh hell broke loose, I had taken Giacomo for his one-year "well-child" checkup. New York State regulations dictated that babies were to be tested for lead at this milestone exam. Our pediatrician neglected to do so. We are white, middle class and college-educated. Perhaps not the "typical" family impacted by lead poisoning. I've often wondered if the doctor's unconscious bias influenced his judgment when he decided not to test Giacomo for lead.

As I reflect on everything that happened, I can't help but ponder the bigger implications of unconscious bias in healthcare. Were there biases that led to an emphasis on beating the cancer over the pain and suffering we'd have to endure as a result of the treatment? Was Jim's relative youth a factor? Did the doctors presume that well-educated, middle-class white people would make the same choices that they themselves would make?

All along our journey down the cancer path, the "risks and side effects" discussion was minimized compared to the heft given to the treatment strategies. In hindsight, I think there should have been an additional consent form that read something like this:

Do you consent to:
- Almost dying anyway because chemo poisons the fuck out of your whole body?
- Feeling sick all the time—like 'teenage hangover with a terrible flu' sick?
- Not being able to eat?
- Bouts of constipation punctuated by unexpected bouts of diarrhea?
- Not being able to do many of the things you like to do, like play music, have sex with your wife, paint, or hike?
- Not being able to do the things you don't like to do like clean the kitchen, shop or mow the lawn?

I wonder how many people would sign that consent form? Would it really be such a bad thing if more people opted out? I don't want to sound like I'm oversimplifying, especially because each cancer has its own complicated biochemistry and each body is different. But it's an important philosophical discussion that the larger community may be avoiding. Perhaps doctors don't paint the full picture because they are driven by a moral imperative to do no harm. But "do no harm" itself is subjective.

As far as I can tell, the only other times people suffer the type of physical pain, anguish and psychological torment that comes with cancer treatments are prison camps and countries where entire populations of people are mercilessly persecuted. The difference is that prisoners and the oppressed don't volunteer for torture, and rarely are they promised that it's being done for their own good.

Another complicating factor in this discussion is that a patient can't truly know what they're going to feel like until they're fully in it. How can you give thoughtful consent to a bunch of *maybes*? During this diagnosis discussion, *prognosis* was never mentioned. We didn't have that TV drama moment where the doctor announces with grave intensity: "You have one month to live." Odds weren't being given on length of life with or without treatment, leaving the biggest "maybe" dangling like a big, gaudy pinata above a bunch of overly eager residents wielding clubs.

We were under an enormous amount of pressure, trying to make an informed decision while dealing with so many unknowns. I think that's why we were only able to focus on the main "live or die?" question. What else do you do when your "Circle of Life" has turned into a roulette wheel? Jim put all his money down on *live* and signed the consent form. Once Jim's decision to proceed was made and the forms were signed, we were left alone to contemplate the larger existential issues at hand. Jim became very quiet as he ventured alone into his thoughts about mortality.

The next day, my sister Diane arrived from Buffalo to check in on us. As a doctor of obstetrics and gynecology, she was familiar with healthcare culture. We relied on her not only as our medical translator, but as the person who could explain things to our family as well. Jim told her he wanted to name her as his second healthcare proxy. This pronouncement opened up a conversation about painful preparatory end-of-life considerations. We were very hopeful, but Jim and I both are practical people. He wanted to make sure certain things were going to be taken care of in case this didn't go the way we all wanted it to. It was a very emotional conversation. The reality of Jim's disease was sinking in. It was hard for all of us to talk about the possibility that he might not beat it.

Because Jim met my sister shortly after he met me back in 1990 when we were all in our 20's, in a way, we all grew up together. As the three of us were talking, crying and sharing a very private and intimate moment, the hospital custodian came in. He took to his job with volume and flourish, as if every task required thespian zeal. I was impressed by the magician-like flare he used to open a new trash bag. I was less impressed by the fact that his excessive clanging and clattering was interrupting our conversation.

As we lowered our voices and huddled closer for privacy, he became louder and more animated. Finally, when he moved in close to aggressively sweep under my feet, I sat back with a "Ok dude. What the fuck do you want?" look on my face. He seized the moment he'd been waiting for, and without any respect for our privacy, he said: "Excuse me. do you all mind if I pray for you?" Stunned by his audacity, I just stared at him, wide-eyed, while an emotionally exhausted Jim uttered: "Sure."

My husband didn't affiliate with any particular faith. For the most part, he thought organized religions were disingenuous. The cancer diagnosis did not alter his perspective. Jim found his peace and a connection to a higher power when he was out in nature. That's what gave him comfort and confidence. He lived his life honestly and simply. He didn't entertain a notion that he needed his relationship with God to be sanctioned by any particular person hawking their religion.

The custodian was a tall man. He stood towering over the foot of Jim's bed, looking like he wasn't going to take no for an answer. I could see Jim's thought process floating in his eyes like clouds. He decided to interpret the intrusion as an act of kindness and allowed the man to carry on with his performance.

Having spent years feeling the heat of my husband's body language when he didn't want me to get into it with anyone (think waiters, salespeople, etc.), I read Jim's vibe and allowed for the imposition. Besides, I don't think either of us could withstand conflict while in our emotionally vulnerable state. I fear it was a calculated manipulation on the part of this uninvited pseudo-cleric.

Now that he had the floor, the custodian's message was delivered more like a lecture than a prayer. There was no raising of hands or bowing of heads. He yammered on about miraculous healings and told Jim that if he asked God for forgiveness and prayed hard, he'd get better.

Ah, the marvelous Health Insurance Portability and Accountability Act (HIPAA) and its promises that you have a right to privacy in your medical care. My suspicions that HIPAA is a charade meant to satisfy bureaucrats rather than actually protect patient privacy were confirmed by this Custodian for Christ. Most of the time HIPAA is just a bureaucratic nuisance. For example, I can't get clarity on my son's doctor bill, which I'm responsible for paying, without my son's signature on a form. Which form? I'm not sure. I print them off as instructed by both the insurance company and the doctor's office. I spend the week hunting down my son for his signature and turn it in only to be told that it isn't the right form. I repeat this ridiculousness several times until the office finally accepts a form. (I picture a *Far Side* cartoon drawing of office administrators huddled around a phone, telling me to go find a different form, then putting themselves on mute so they can laugh their asses off while I react.)

But this "patient privacy" regulation somehow does not cover a doctor yelling a life-altering cancer diagnosis to my husband in a hospital hallway that's as busy as Penn Station at rush hour for everyone in a one-mile radius to hear (which, in this case, was about a thousand people). Or a custodian interrupting a personal end-of-life conversation to proselytize.

After the three-minute sermon about miracles and forgiveness ended, we proceeded with a hushed and muted version of our conversation. Our privacy having been invaded, we now felt like we were being listened to and judged. I told one of the nurses what happened. She responded sheepishly with: "He shouldn't be doing that." *Oh gee, ya think?* I was furious. Jim, on the other hand, was in a different frame of mind. He was way past his capacity to handle any more tension. During the days leading up to this incident, the custodian had been affable and pleasant—personality traits Jim appreciated like a cool glass of water on a hot day. Though Jim wasn't about to "ask for forgiveness," he was definitely ready to dispense it liberally. My job as his wife was to support a tranquil environment as best I could. It would have been a dereliction of duty if I'd made a scene with our crusading custodian.

In the wake of Jim's passing, I've come to realize that a large part of my trauma stems from the fact that we were deeply violated. Not by any one person, but by the whole process. The entire cancer experience from start to finish managed to violate our family physically, psychologically, emotionally, and spiritually. What happens to your mind when you consent to torture? This trespass hasn't been acknowledged in a meaningful way. Nor, do I expect, will it ever be, because the cancer industry is normalized by our culture.

Cancer therapies are a series of acts of violence. Cognitively, you consent because it's the only option that might give you a shot at staying alive. But choosing to pursue treatment means you acquiesce to brutal assaults until one day you either reach remission, cure, or death. And cure is not a path to the "self" you knew minutes before your diagnosis. The cancer survivor is permanently altered mentally and physically.

Though your intellect follows what the doctors are saying and sort of understands the logic of the options, the rest of your body and mind aren't so sure about what's in the offing. Consent is only granted by your higher-order executive function, leaving the rest of your psyche to grapple with the fallout. That's why coping with the violence is so difficult and confusing. What exacerbates the trauma is the silence around its perpetration. No one expresses chest thumping outrage. There isn't even a fist pump to righteous indignation. People move around the cancer center offering limp "I know this is a lot" and "I'm so sorry you're going through this." The sentiments don't even come close to matching the egregiousness of cancer treatments.

Modern medicine relies on a few therapies for cancer treatment. There is a growing body of research into new methods like immunotherapies. But for now, the aggressive poisoning of your body with chemotherapy and radiation often accompanied by butchering surgery remain the preferred (dare I say lucrative?) treatment options. As a result, the brutality is normalized by our medical community and accepted by our society.

With Jim's consent in hand, the oncologist's goal was to keep Jim's body alive. Between treatments, the rest of the team was tasked with managing the physical fallout from the aggressive therapies. However, the team turned a blind eye to the mental and emotional anguish suffered by Jim and his family. (More on this later.) It seemed the doctors and nurses in the cancer center had developed their own emotional buffers to help them cope with walking the tight rope over death canyon every day. I certainly don't begrudge them their coping skills. They needed to be able to focus their medical minds on solving the problems of the diseases their patients endured. I can't even imagine what it's like to experience death as a regular part of one's job. If they didn't have some way of coping, they'd never be able to function. Still, I couldn't help but feel that the disconnect between the torrent of emotions we were feeling and the healthcare team's clinical approach to Jim's care unintentionally became a form of gaslighting. As if everything was normal.

When we walked into the hospital, Jim had to surrender his privacy, his dignity, and his personhood in exchange for an army that would fight his disease. A psychological shift took place in him almost immediately upon diagnosis. He quickly developed his own emotional buffer in order to participate in the war. This must be how he was able to convince himself to acquiesce to the treatment while also grappling with end-of-life considerations. My normally feisty husband adopted a demur and compliant demeanor. Cancer has a sinister way of humbling the mighty.

Jim always used to say "There are worse things than death." Usually, he'd make this statement after we watched a particularly disturbing news report or a documentary about WWII. In the months that followed his diagnosis, he lived the actualization of that sentiment.

CHAPTER SIX

Forty Days in the Hole

Day six was marked by great relief for everyone. Jim was being released from the ICU, back into the care of the cancer center. (Oddly, for the second time in one week, the cancer center was a step up from where we were.) Jim's body cooperated with the interventions that slowly brought him back from the "critical condition" cliff. The initial treatments were doing their job to hold off the advancing mob of lymphoblasts, allowing improved blood oxygenation. Jim still needed the nose cannoli for oxygen support (it's actually called a cannula, but cannoli is more fun to say), but that was much less invasive and threatening than the Darth Vader helmet.

Our first week in the hospital was fraught with the frantic energy born of sheer panic. If I could assign a sound to the colliding cultures of "healthy, normal life at home" with "terminal illness in a hospital," it would be a deafening explosion of metal and glass. Though our ears were still ringing from the initial explosion, we soldiered on and set to the task of assessing the damage and preparing for the ensuing war.

Test results eliminated any ambiguity. We had a known foe. We also had a dedicated coach, team, arsenal of weaponry, and a strategy, designed to vanquish our adversary. Though the disease was rare, we were fortunate (in a relative sense) that our oncologist was knowledgeable about T-cell ALL. She told us she consulted regularly with a national group of doctors who focused on the various treatments, therapies, and clinical trials for adult T-cell ALL. She was a formidable coach indeed.

With the most critical aspects of Jim's illness temporarily under control, it was now time for us to focus on driving this beast of a cancer into remission. We were mentally preparing ourselves for four weeks of in-patient chemotherapy. After our sobering conversation with Dr. B, we realized we had another difficult task ahead of us. Whether we wanted to or not, we had to share the news of Jim's condition.

We live in Rochester, NY—a midsized city where news travels fast. I wasn't concerned about the grapevine broadcasting Jim's illness. As long as our immediate family heard directly from us, then the grapevine was going to be a useful tool. The issue we faced was traffic control for the subsequent outpouring. My husband was a good man who was kind and generous of spirit. He came from a large family and had an incredible universe of friends.

There's something about saying the words "I have leukemia" out loud that solidifies the painful reality. Having to say them repeatedly is akin to stabbing yourself in the thigh with a steak knife over and over again. Fielding people's reactions and responses to your news makes it even more emotionally trying. Frankly, trying to cope with how others reacted was very difficult for me. I still don't have the capacity for it. Amazingly, the patient did a much better job handling it than I did.

The pain of it all wasn't our only reason for minimizing these conversations. We needed to focus on Jim and everything that was happening in our immediate surroundings. He needed rest in between his trips through the gauntlet that was chemotherapy.

The first order of business was a conversation with Jim's boss. He couldn't just call in sick. The doctor didn't think Jim would be able to go back to work for at least a year, which meant he would have to file for disability. Next, we had the very difficult task of telling Jim's mother, Rose. She was 90 years old and in pretty decent health. She'd survived her husband and all six of her siblings. Three of her sisters died from cancer, and in 90 years, she'd seen many friends lose ugly fights with "the big C". She knew full well what devastation accompanied a cancer diagnosis.

At 56 years of age, Jimmy was still her baby. Telling her that Jim had cancer was going to be absolutely brutal. Jim called his brother Frank and sister Kathy to give them the news. They agreed to be at Rose's house when Jim called so they could be there for support. Ugh. She was absolutely distraught. Her post-traumatic stress from watching so many loved ones die from cancer was fully triggered. She sobbed and wanted to come to the hospital immediately. Understandable.

My parents needed an update as well. My sister Diane was already with us for much of the first week. Like Jim's siblings, she laid the groundwork with my parents, but I still needed to call them. I knew they'd be upset and very worried.

With the job and family notifications done, I wanted to find a way to manage the communication with the rest of our universe so it was effective, not overwhelming. I knew we were going to get inundated with calls and texts that we weren't in a position to handle. Hell, I couldn't find my car in the parking lot. How could I actually talk to people? At the same time, Jim was definitely going to need support. I wanted him to be accessible in a healthy way so he could feel the love and encouragement. My hand needed to be on the throttle so he was buoyed by the well wishes, not drowned by them. Fortunately, I remembered a website a friend used several years ago to post information about his progress when he was struggling with illness. I did a quick internet search for the site when the calls started coming in. CaringBridge was the first website to pop up in my search. A cursory view proved the site was going to be the answer to my communication prayers. CaringBridge's nonprofit status means they don't run ads or sell user data, unlike the Metaverse. This was the perfect user-friendly tool I needed to disseminate information quickly. I signed up for an account right away.

Late at night, I'd write my entries in the CaringBridge journal like it was my diary. The dimmed hospital lights and low hum of machines lulled my excited mind into a temporary peace where I could sort through the day's events. Conveying our story in this format helped me unwind what was happening so I could plan for the next day. The responses to my posts were deeply moving. It felt like I was having a private conversation with each person. Through CaringBridge, loved ones from far and wide kept me company and gave me strength to keep fighting the fight.

Jim didn't read the entries himself. Sometimes he would want me to read them aloud, but most of the time, he chose to skip it when I offered. He was living it. He didn't need my play-by-play. People commented to him frequently about how much they enjoyed the posts. He would share all the feedback with me and say: "You're such a good writer! I've always said you should write." (He was my biggest cheerleader.) When he was emotionally able to tolerate them, I would read Jim the comments. The messages of love and encouragement were so touching, he'd become overwhelmed with emotion. When I saw him get misty-eyed and retreat inwards, I'd stop reading to give him time to process.

CHAPTER SEVEN

Hospital Life

Getting used to living in a hospital wasn't easy. I had to rethink all aspects of my daily routine, from eating to parking the car. For example, from the very first trip to the emergency room, finding my car in the hospital's six-tiered parking garage made me feel like a contestant on a game show. I was so upset and overwhelmed, I forgot where I parked every single time. I would spend a minimum of 15 minutes every day, running up and down the stairs, wandering around parking levels, pressing my key fob and listening for my Jeep. I'm sure I had a vacant look on my face while seemingly walking in circles. If someone watched a recording of my parking garage promenades, they would likely make the assumption that I had escaped from the memory care unit. In the early days of Jim's diagnosis, I would make a mental note of the floor level color and number of my space, committing the information to memory with confidence and certitude. Alas, when I returned, it was like I just arrived from Mars and didn't even know what a car was.

During my many scavenger hunts around the garage, I observed the public's entertaining parking strategies used to meet the challenges presented by the curious parking ramp design. The angled spaces were too close together. Even if you parked perfectly between the lines (which was hard to do because it only took one person parking over one line to completely throw off an entire row), the likelihood of being able to open your car door enough to extricate your entire body in one try was slim. And heaven forfend you had any bags with you. I had to climb into my driver's seat from the passenger side more times than you could imagine. I'm a petite person. I don't know how your average-sized adult did it.

To some degree, my parking aggravations were diffused by the friendly parking lot attendants. During the day, I'd bottle up all my fears and sadness. It only took one parking attendant's sincere "Have a good afternoon!" on my way out of the garage to uncork all my tears. But their stellar customer service wasn't enough to prevent me from becoming obsessed with the poor lot design. I literally took pictures of the parking spots and wonky parking jobs and measured my parking spaces with a tape measure to figure out the math for how one was supposed to open their car door all the way in order to get in and out. I was going to send a letter to management. It blows my mind that the designers of the lot thought their spacing would work for anyone other than a ballet dancer driving a Mini Cooper. I know, I know. Totally cuckoo. After all the physical and emotional strain of our cancer life in the hospital, ruminating over the parking garage puzzle solve was a sedating mental task. Almost like playing one of those handheld pinball games I had when I was a kid.

Two weeks into our stay, I finally had the presence of mind to park on the garage's rooftop level. There were multiple benefits to this strategy. First, I always knew where my car was.

Second, it wasn't considered an optimal location because your car would be exposed to the elements, so I was assured a good spot. Often, I was one of the few cars up there so I didn't have to climb in through the trunk or worry about my car getting dinged. Lastly, I could see Jim's room from where I parked. I could call him when I arrived or when I was leaving and wave to him. I'd often do some kind of silly dance to make him laugh. (I later realized that the construction workers on the floor underneath him could also see me dance. I should've taken the opportunity to flip them off for waking him up all the time with their stupid power tools.) This was like my secret, VIP parking space. Garage management plowed well and regularly, so I never had to worry about getting snowed in.

Once the chaos of our first week settled down, we got into a rhythm with our treatment plan and succumbed, albeit begrudgingly, to hospital life. In the beginning, Jim did pretty well. His body tolerated the chemo better than we both expected. He looked so good! You'd never guess he was a patient. As I mentioned earlier, he grew his beard out, perhaps in anticipation of losing his hair. One last hirsute "hoorah," if you will. The chemo would give him the standard nausea and fatigue, but he bounced back from the first few treatments relatively quickly. His tolerance of the treatments nurtured our optimism.

When he was feeling up to it, he'd talk or text on his phone with friends and read or draw. People suggested we bring in things from home to help Jim feel more comfortable, but he didn't want his things. We were in agreement on this point. We did not want to engage in some depressing attempt to somehow morph Jim's hospital room into a sad version of our bedroom. The hospital was decidedly *not* our home. And *going home* was a goal that gave Jim a sense of purpose. The only item he really wanted was his mandolin. He didn't play it much, but he found it comforting to have in his possession nonetheless. As luck would have it, one of his nurses was a musician. Nurse M brought in his guitar so they could play together during his breaks. They'd talk about the Rochester music scene and play a tune or two. Jim enjoyed Nurse M's company and I appreciated his genuine interest in Jim as a person, not a patient. Playing with Nurse M took the performance pressure off Jim. If his bandmates came in to play, they'd notice his declining abilities. Nurse M had never heard Jim play, so he had nothing to compare him to and, as an oncology nurse, he was eager to celebrate the musician that Jim was at heart.

Although Jim chose visual art for his profession, his creativity didn't stop there. He had a passion for music that he expressed in his younger years through the acoustic guitar. Back in the days before children, we caroused at festivals and parties that revolved around home-made music. Memories of mirth-filled nights spent singing and dancing with our friends until the roosters told us it was time to settle down glow in my heart like the bonfires we sat around. At home, we enjoyed playing together as a couple. He'd accompany me on the guitar while I sang. Those were special times—like the world was on hold while we created together.

Playing with our musician friends whet Jim's appetite for more opportunities to perform. Though he enjoyed the guitar, he was in search of a broader musical experience. Forever a student of his heritage, he'd been listening to Italian folk music where the mandolin figured prominently. My auditory line was crossed the day Jim came home with a CD of Italian fishermen singing old folk songs. When he pressed "play", this horrible noise emanated from the speakers—like a kraken yodeling. That's when I decided to scrape my pennies together and buy him a mandolin.

Saving money wasn't the hard part. Shopping for a musical instrument that I knew nothing about was the challenge. And Jim was a lefty, which complicated matters. Internet shopping wasn't as prevalent then, but I think that actually simplified my search. I made a couple phone calls and as luck would have it, I found the only left-handed mandolin in the area at a music store across town. The boys and I were delighted to present this gift to him for Father's Day. The instrument was a little beat up, and I had no idea if it was any good, but none of that mattered to Jim because it was love at first sight. The mandolin opened up a whole new world of music for him and eventually set him down his path to becoming a bona fide gig musician.

Once the instrument was in his hot hands, he spent hours learning how to play. He took a few lessons here and there, but it was the guys who eventually became his bandmates that taught him the most. String Theory, their bluegrass band, got off the ground in the early 2000's. They developed their sound as they played weddings and town festivals. Eventually, they landed a weekly gig at a local bar. Both Jim's musicianship and management skills strengthened over time. I'm not sure if it was because Jim was the most motivated or the most organized, but he ended up managing the business side to keep the very thirsty band cash-positive.

While Jim's love of live music blossomed, mine waned. Sadly, it wasn't something we enjoyed as a couple anymore. The kids were young, so while he was out chasing his dream, I was home chasing little boys. The early years of parenting were filled with high-energy, nonstop activity. In a word?

Exhausting. I would bring the kids to some of the gigs, but it was more work than it was worth. If I managed to hire a babysitter, I'd be stuck in the audience with a bunch of drunks who'd blather on about the band members of "Phish" like my kids talked about Pokémon characters. Instead of watching my husband, my eyes were on the clock because we couldn't afford the babysitter for much more than two hours.

When the kids were in elementary school, I did a cannonball into the deep end of the workforce by taking a job with the governor's office. Staffer jobs can be thankless, 24/7 meat grinders. When I wasn't at work, my mind was on high alert for the next knee-jerk, panic directive from the "second floor," the locus of power in New York State. Many stay-at-home moms who rejoin the workforce will appreciate the manic approach I took to proving my value after being home with my children for seven years. I was no longer as present as I should've been for our family. Shortly after I started my new position, Jim got laid off from his job. In an instant, our roles were reversed. Jim became a stay-at-home dad, while developing his own freelance graphic design business. His new status aggravated his fear of being broke, so he was on the hunt for more gigs to supplement our income.

It took me a while to pull my head out of my own low self-esteem issues to realize that the layoff had a big impact on Jim's psyche. His identity as a professional and as a provider had been called into question, shaking his sense of value and purpose. He was left to face the hobgoblins of money worries, shame and depression while keeping a stiff upper lip in the court of public opinion. Let's face it, back then, the only people who looked favorably on stay-at-home dads were a man's wife and kids.

Our individual dynamism brought complexity to our relationship. While Jim continued to nurture his thirst for musical experiences, I became a workaholic at a job I thought mattered. We fed our obsessive ambitions while holding fast to our deeply rooted family values. It doesn't take a genius to see how our situation would be ripe for conflict. Jim and I loved each other fiercely—that was the easy part. The hard part was relationshipping. Collaborating on parenting, home ownership, career directions and money management while coping with the surprise stressors that pounce out of life's bag o' tricks at times felt Sisyphean. The most well-adjusted marriages can steer off course when they enter the Bermuda triangle of Me. You. Us. Ours was no different.

Though the waters were choppy, I don't want to give you the impression that it was a constant storm. I suppose when you talk about the deeper hardships of a relationship that aren't typically shared at a cocktail party, one might jump to the conclusion that we were headed for disaster. I view it as the normal rough and tumble of living a full life. We continued to parent, to work on our relationship, and to build our lives together. We never stopped loving each other, so we persevered through the toughest parts. In fact, I think that's what frustrated us the most. As we ran by each other, we built walls between us that were making it increasingly more difficult to communicate in a way that supported a healthy relationship.

The "band" wall was probably our biggest obstacle, eventually dividing us like 1961 Germany. I viewed Jim's amateur music career as an aggressive intrusion on our family time. When the band hit their stride, they were playing out a couple of nights during the week. Weddings sucked up Saturdays and an additional night was dedicated to practice.

Factor in the time it takes to travel places, load equipment, set up and break down—you've got a pretty significant time commitment. When I complained, which was often, he'd point out the fact that he was bringing an additional income into the household. My response was something cruel like: "Let's face it, you're not the Rolling Stones. What you're making isn't worth the time it's taking away from us." As Jim added instruments, gigs and different bands to his repertoire, my resentment approached the boiling point. My proud memories of gifting him his first mandolin were replaced with fantasies of smashing the shit out of it on the sidewalk in front of our house.

I was torn because I wanted him to enjoy what he loved doing. But somehow, it seemed more like escapism than a healthy hobby. The fact that he unapologetically managed to book a gig on our wedding anniversary every single year made me wonder if he was being pulled by music or pushing away from me? Eventually I realized that much of Jim's identity after he lost his job was attached to his view of himself as a musician. It stands to reason that my criticisms and protests were received as a rejection. And when your partner is rejecting the very thing that validates your self-worth, then why would you want to spend time with them?

Things came to a head when the boys were starting high school. I told Jim that my patience had worn thin and that I was tired of taking the backseat to his musical aspirations. I wanted my husband back and if I couldn't have him, then I wanted out of our marriage. Frankly, my pronouncement was sobering to the both of us. Once the words were out of my mouth, I knew that wasn't what I wanted, but it was the only thing I could think of to get Jim's attention. Something about the shock factor opened a door for us to have a meaningful conversation, free from the white noise of useless bickering. Rather than blaming Jim for everything, I started to openly admit that I brought a wheelbarrow—maybe two—full of garbage to our marital bonfire. My admission softened Jim's defensive position. We stopped the blame game foes engage in and regrouped as a couple. Step by step, day by day, we started deconstructing the walls we built around our hearts, and reinventing our relationship in a way that satisfied us both.

Weight training creates microtears in your muscle fibers. When your body is at rest between weight lifting sessions, it sends reinforcements to heal the microtears. The soreness you feel is a sign that the repair process is working. Over time, that repeated process of tearing and healing strengthens and builds your muscles. I view that contentious period in our lives as our weight training regimen for our relationship. We worked our way through it with our clumsy, self-taught conflict resolution skills while spotting each other to keep the family ship afloat. Though it sucked, I think our "tearing and repairing" process is what made our marital partnership as strong as Tungsten. I'm so grateful to Jim and proud of us both for reaching that sweet spot in our relationship. Those last six years together felt like our first six.

CHAPTER EIGHT

Settling in

While he was poked, prodded and poisoned around the clock by countless people, I was trying to hold on to some shred of dignity for both of us. From a morale perspective, I didn't want him to *look* like a patient, so I tried to get him to wear a T-shirt and pants, for example. But the room temperature was inconsistent and his clothes had to come off so many times for different procedural reasons that shorts became the preferred attire. Which meant he was half naked most of the time. It drove me crazy as his room was a revolving door of strangers. His emotional buffer served him well because he didn't seem to mind. He remained sociable and kind with everyone throughout his entire stay.

There was a privacy curtain that ran the width of the room when you first walked in because the double doors had large windows in them. There were no restrictions on visitors, so all kinds of people were walking the hallways. People were respectful, but still, you don't want to be on display in your birthday suit as people walked by. Thus, the privacy curtain. Because there was a lot of up and down in various stages of wellness and dress, I kept the curtain closed. Not all of the staff were as mindful of the privacy aspect. Some days it was like an annoying game: I'd close the curtain; someone would come in and whip it open, perform their task, then depart. I'd get up and close the curtain again; repeat. Annoying.

Daily walks through our neighborhood were an activity we enjoyed at home, so we just continued our regimen in the hospital. It was a seamless transition for us to go from enjoying the different architectural styles and murals in our city neighborhood, to taking in the artwork adorning the halls of the medical center and commenting on the various departmental office designs. You wouldn't think it, but a hospital is fun to explore, with all its nooks and crannies and constant activity. It has the feel of a mini city.

Spending that kind of time together was precious. Jim was such a good conversationalist. After 30 years together, I enjoyed his company as much as I did when I first fell in love with him. He always had interesting thoughts and ideas about the world around us that challenged me to think deeper. Jim's knowledge about art and art history was encyclopedic, making him the best art gallery companion. His thoughtful perspective made viewing the hospital collection livelier and much more interesting than if I were viewing it alone.

When he was feeling good, we'd make the hospital rounds twice a day. We liked to see how the departments were set up and joked that we should hang out in every waiting room to sample the coffee and rate the "patient experience," like Yelp reviewers. We'd browse around the gift shop and go to the cafeteria for an ice cream. He'd indulge my ridiculous addiction to decaf coffee, waiting for me while I stood in line at the coffee cart. Often, we'd see some of his doctors and nurses in our travels, waving "Hello." We were engaged in an entirely different "Who are the people in your neighborhood?" experience, but it satisfied our need for exercise and human contact.

Our favorite places to visit were the children's hospital and the chapel. The décor in the children's hospital was bright and cheery. The entryway had a vaulted ceiling and big windows. We actually learned how to properly wash a window by watching the service in action. We chatted with one of the window washers about the technique and where to buy the equipment. He was very friendly and told us all about the process. I think he appreciated someone genuinely taking an interest in his work.

There was a second entrance to the Children's hospital that had a cool tropical fish tank in the foyer. Someone crafted several colorful models of fish that appeared as an extension of the aquarium on the hall walls. They were whimsical and fun. Sometimes when Jim was especially tired, we'd sit in one of the waiting rooms surrounded by toys and zone out to children's television programming. Though we were clearly out of place, the staff never objected to our loitering. Maybe Jim looked sicker than I thought.

The chapel was tucked away from the hustle and bustle of the hospital, providing a much-appreciated buffer between us and the tension of infirmity. We visited at all hours and never found it locked. I was glad to learn that the gods don't keep strict visiting hours. The spiritual atmosphere offered solace as we sat in contemplative silence together. I never asked Jim what he was thinking about while we were in the chapel. In hindsight, I realize it was a missed opportunity for us to open up to each other about our fears and sadness. There we were, sitting on the lip of eternity's maw, staring into the abyss. As painful as it might have been, talking about death could have soothed us and brought us closer. Maybe we could have even injected some wonder into our hearts at the awesome mystery of life. Regrettably, I let my worries hold the silent space between us.

In front of Jim, I maintained an administrative demeanor by managing his care coordination. I'd take notes, make lists, keep track of people and medicines with fervor. There was a glorious amount of busy work for someone who didn't want to sit with her feelings or just spend time looking into her husband's eyes. I didn't let Jim see that his death was haunting me. I was afraid admitting my fears would sound defeatist, thereby negatively impacting his will to fight the disease. You hear people talk about setting intentions and staying positive while they're critically ill. In my opinion, there's an overemphasis on positive thinking in our culture—as if you can magically wish your cancer away. Maybe it's just me, but folks who promote the "positive attitude" prescription seem to deliver their philosophy on a plate made of judgement. Frankly, I think that attitude is bullshit, because it shames people who don't feel "positive" about their illness and dissuades them from engaging in real conversations about what it means to die. Exploring those thoughts and feelings is difficult emotional work, but it's much more authentic than whistling a happy tune and hiding behind phony sentiment. I avoided certain friends who were inclined to promote the "power of positive thinking" crap because I was miserable and didn't have the wherewithal to pretend otherwise. It amazes me that we as humans are able to contemplate end of life, but we still haven't found a way to cope with the natural fact that death happens.

Maybe I'm so annoyed by the adverse relationship between positive thinking and our realism because I'm embarrassed and angry with myself for putting my emotions on the back burner while I was with Jim. Late February, I finally cried in front of him while we were talking to one of his doctors. Jim looked at me and with surprise in his voice, said "That's the first time I've seen you get upset." I realized that preventing myself from dissolving into an emotional puddle deprived my husband of the feels he was craving. He wanted to know—needed to know—that his wife was heartbroken because that's the right feeling to have if you love someone who is suffering. I was startled and ashamed by the realization that my "all business" approach to Jim's care was hurting his feelings. But even after that exchange, I don't think I did a good enough job of sharing my pain and sadness. Maybe I was afraid of not being able to collect myself to continue providing care. Or—perhaps with reason—I feared that the doctors wouldn't take me seriously. Sitting in the pain was both excruciating and necessary for both of us, but my conscious mind couldn't do it. God, I hate myself sometimes.

All of our activity was punctuated by nurses and nurse assistants distributing medications, taking vitals, checking urine output, etc. The dietitians would leapfrog the nurses throughout the day to collect Jim's meal orders. They were as good-natured as they were efficient. If Jim was indecisive or if he wasn't feeling well, the dieticians would wait patiently and remind him of all the kitchen's offerings. They got to know Jim's preferences throughout his chemo cycles so they could make informed a la carte suggestions when he wasn't up for choosing a whole meal. I imagine talking to chemo patients every day wore on their souls, but they never, not once, displayed impatience or frustration. They added a drop of normalcy to our days because the transaction had a hint of diner waitress about it.

Our family always loved a good diner. For years we referred to the Greek diner in our neighborhood as our second kitchen. We have countless memories of eating there as a family. They should've named a booth after us. If I ran out of ideas, patience, or food, we all packed in the car and went to Gitsis. When the boys hit their remarkable food consumption stride in high school, they would order two entrees each to sate their voracious appetites. Despite the fact that we were ordering everything on the menu in one sitting, we could still afford the check. All the waitresses were friendly, fast, and fierce. When the boys were little, the diner was open 24/7, serving the unruly Monroe Avenue bar crowd until the wee hours of the morning. The waitresses had to pull double duty as bouncers. Late-night Monroe Avenue was a completely different scene than daytime Monroe Avenue.

One of Gianni's kindergarten teachers asked him where he liked to eat as part of a "getting to know you" exercise. He enthusiastically replied "Gitsis!". She was stunned at first, then burst out laughing. I imagine her only Gitsis reference was based on the hazy vision of one who frequented the local bars before filling up on eggs and bacon. It didn't occur to her that regular families ate there during the day, so her shock at Gianni's favorite place was genuine, albeit naïve. An image of my little five-year-old Gianni swaggering into Gitsis at three a.m. wearing a biker jacket and an air of kick-ass makes me laugh too. Sadly, one too many late-night ruckuses shut the diner down. We were all deeply saddened by the closing of our second kitchen. The boys and I still search Rochester like culinary nomads for a suitable replacement.

Jim perked right up when the dietitians came in. He was as good an eater as he was a talker, so the waitress-like feel from the dietitians coupled with the promise of food temporarily took Jim's mind off his illness. The only thing I knew about chemo before we were in the thick of our experience was that cancer patients lose their appetites and their hair. I was somewhat surprised to find that, for the most part, Jim kept his appetite throughout his hospital stay. He'd eat the hospital food, then he'd eat what our friends made him, then I'd run out and grab something from one of the many fast-food places in the area. I believe the steroids contributed to his ability to keep pace with his normal food intake.

Cooking for Jim had always been a satisfying experience. He ate like a goat, which, as the person preparing his meals, you could take a couple of ways. The negative view would be that your cooking wasn't special to someone who would eat sh** if you put it in front of them. I chose the positive view that everything I made was delicious. The truth fell somewhere in between. The digestive prowess of my husband was legendary—and sometimes embarrassing. I remember being invited to my boss's house for dinner in the early '90s. The hostess got up from the table to put something in the refrigerator. In the process, she pulled out a plate of chicken. Jim's face lit up as he exclaimed: "Ooh! Chicken!" It turned out dinner was over. Our hostess was putting food back in the fridge and needed to make room by moving what turned out to be their leftovers from another night. The moment she realized that Jim was still hungry and eyeing what was likely their lunch for the next day coincided with the moment Jim and I realized that he made an exuberant faux pas. There was an embarrassment standoff that ended with a gracious offering of the chicken. Turns out, he wasn't that embarrassed because he ate the chicken. This is a man who actually got kicked out of an "all you can eat" buffet.

Family dinner was an important part of our day. When the kids were school-aged, we gathered almost every night without the distraction of a television, phones, or even music. Consistency was the only formal part of our evening meal. In fact, I'm reluctant to even call it "dinner" because the word suggests a level of dignity wherein people sit around a well-appointed table discussing Chaucer while savoring a splendid meal. Dinner in our house was utter mayhem marked by the inhalation of food in a rush to make sure that you got to eat what was on your plate before the others finished theirs and started in on yours like a pack of wolves. I'm convinced Gianni continued to eat with his hands way past the developmental stage in which one learns to use utensils because it gave him a speed advantage.

This caveman-like behavior was accompanied by banter that was irreverent, offensive and profoundly silly. The boys had a gift for honing in on whatever topic lived at the edges of inappropriate. The three males in my house were constantly trying to outdo each other, pushing the "shock factor" boundaries in order to make each other laugh. The only subjects off limits were the type that would curb an appetite—like explicit details of a nasty bowel movement. That was saved for car talk. Over the years, I recall watching accomplished people regale talk show hosts with their memories of debating current events and discussing the works of leading authors around the dinner table with their families. These stories made me feel we were failing as parents because we weren't leading erudite conversations for the intellectual benefit of our kids. Later in life I realized how phony that would have been for us and how such an attempt would've provoked our sons to display even worse behavior. What dinner lacked in civility, we made up for with mirth. So what if we didn't expand their intellectual horizons every night at the table? We taught them how to be present for one another: to listen to stories from the day, blow off steam, and enjoy a good laugh.

As Jim's nausea ebbed and flowed, we did our best to observe the formality of meal times in our never-ending attempt to normalize our life in the hospital. The boys joined in when their school schedules allowed, injecting a lively chatter that distracted us from our predicament. Hospital dinner time wasn't as robust as our home routine, but it was enough to evoke the memory of a ritual that we all held dear.

Before we turned in for the night, we would watch a show or two. Hospital television was terrible so we used an HDMI cable to hook our computers up to the TV in order to access our streaming services. Comedies were usually on the docket. The boys often joined us, since they were free most evenings. I remember *The Office* was one of our main "go-tos" because it was a show all four of us could agree on. My sister told me we should watch the episode about the fire drill—that it was the funniest thing she'd ever seen. We were all excited to reap the benefits of the best medicine. Just as the show started, a nurse came in to do evening vitals checks and medicine distribution. "Oh! You're watching The Office! I love this show! It's so great your sons are here to watch with you. This is the funniest episode. I love it when the..." (proceeds to spoil the element of surprise that is comedic genius and yammer through the entire scene.) You can't really kick someone out while they're doing important and necessary things to your body. We had to pause and go back after she finally shut up and left.

After the boys left, I'd make up the hospital futon and shut off the main lights. Lights were always shining in from the hallway and blinking from the machines, so it was never totally dark. I'd start out curled up next to Jim in his hospital bed, but it was hard to stay there because it offered few comfortable positions for me. I pretzeled myself around him to keep clear of the wires and tubes. There were awkward interruptions throughout the night as technicians came in to take his vitals and distribute medicines. I wanted Jim to get as much sleep as possible, so I eventually moved to the futon. I'd stay up watching shows or writing on CaringBridge while Jim slept. Most of the time, I was so wired I would just stare out the window and listen to the comings and goings of the Mercy Flight helicopters.

I spent almost every night with Jim. The room was spacious by hospital standards. If the privacy curtain was closed when you first walked in, you could almost imagine the space was a formal entrance into a foyer with a coat closet on the left wall and a utility sink and cupboard to the right. Once past the curtain, you were facing the side of Jim's hospital bed. Medical equipment surrounded the head of Jim's bed to the right. A beautiful picture of a flower hovered above that electrical tangle on the wall above, acting as a calming counterweight to all the flashing bleeps and blips of the equipment. On the wall across from the foot of the bed was a white board on which the nurses wrote important information, like the date, names of the shift nurse and the attending doctors, and important procedures or tests scheduled for the day. There was a mounted television up high on that same wall and below the TV were two cork strips. We tacked up the colorful greeting cards from friends and family on the cork so they were in full, cheery view at all times. In a corner to the right of the TV was a small table with two chairs. This is where we ate our meals. The room extended into a nook-like living area. The nook was equipped with a hospital recliner and the aforementioned futon, neither of which was cushy, but proved adequate. The futon faced the sizeable bathroom. The room ended at a large window that extended from the ceiling, covering three quarters of the wall. From the window, we had a good view of Mt. Hope Cemetery.

One might think a graveyard would be a terrible view for a cancer patient. However, Mt. Hope has a country charm about its landscaping that speaks more of life than death. Established in 1838 as the country's first municipal cemetery, Mt. Hope is graced with majestic trees and winding paths that invite contemplation. There are over 350,000 people buried there. You'd think they'd cause a commotion every now and again, but as far as I know, they've never thrown a rave. Our family spent countless hours over the years enjoying walks through this community gem. Though we weren't in our home, the view of the cemetery was a daily reminder that we were in our neighborhood. Gazing out the window, we felt a serenity born of familiarity.

The nurses tried to make me as comfortable as possible, continually offering sheets, blankets and pillows. Though sleeping in the hospital felt more like glamping, I appreciated the accommodations and their kindness. They made me feel welcome, unlike my time in the maternity ward with newborn Gianni.

In the afternoons, after the rounding docs came through, I'd run home to do laundry, pick up food, take a shower, sort myself out and repack for the next 24 hours. Both entrance and egress were marked by my Sherpa impersonation. On the way out, I'd lug my backpack and a bag in each hand. My backpack contained my computer, notebooks and reading material. The bags were filled with empty food containers and Jim's laundry. Upon my return, the bags were filled with fresh food, clean duds and more cards and gifts from friends.

In my mind, the cancer belonged to both of us. It stood to reason that fighting it was our fulltime job. Everything I did was in service of our goal to achieve remission. When I wasn't in the hospital, I was cleaning, shopping, doing laundry, researching, and coordinating. It never occurred to me to do anything else. Being unemployed eliminated any hard decisions I'd have to make about time vis-à-vis Jim's care. If I had been working full time, I'm not sure how I would have managed.

Throughout Jim's illness, I craved a physical closeness with him. I wanted to climb inside his body and use my immune system to help fight his disease. It may sound like a no-brainer for a spouse to want to stand by their sick partner, but the truth is, the pain of helplessly watching your loved one suffer is intolerable. Despite the agonizing helplessness I felt, it never occurred to me to be anywhere else but in the trenches with him.

I supervised his care with an intense vigilance because I was desperate to see signs of improvement. At times, Jim's judgment was cloudy. Whether it was the medicines, lack of sleep, or preoccupation with the existential crisis of dying, his mental acuity wasn't always 100%. Acting as his onsite advocate, I was able to fill in the blanks for the doctors and backstop anything that might have slipped through the cracks of a busy ward.

CHAPTER NINE

Friends and Family

Jim was one of the first of his contemporaries to be victimized by a life-threatening illness. What amplified the surprise was that he was likely the healthiest among them. The news sent a shockwave through our friend groups. I can only imagine the middle-aged angst the news provoked, driving many to gaze fearfully into their mirrors, begging answerless questions about purpose and mortality.

Outside the hospital walls, our nation was on edge. Political discourse wallowed in a dark place, pitting family members and friends against each other. Rancor was being sprayed generously over our country through the manure spreader that is social media. Reports of a virus spreading in Asia faintly foreshadowed the pandemic, adding a heightened level of unease to this scenario.

Once Jim's illness was broadcast, we received a tie-dye rainbow of emotional responses from family and friends. Primarily, we were the beneficiaries of unbridled expressions of love. Battalions of people sent cards, gifts, emails, texts, art, poems, and food. Our people were incredibly generous throughout our struggle. Countless messages conveying heartfelt sentiments of love, faith, and support buoyed our spirits and warmed our hearts. Reading the cards and tacking them up on the wall across from Jim's bed so he could see and feel the collective support from his well-wishers was a daily event, brightening our shaded days. Our friends let us know continually how loved we were and that we weren't alone. The notes kept us in touch with the healthy world outside the confines of the hospital. These expressions of raw, stripped-down love have been tattooed on my soul and continue to warm my heart like an eternal flame.

Often, I found myself in a position of trying to convince people that their cards, emails, and texts were impactful. I suppose it feels minimal to send a card to someone who is so sick. "Surely, there must be something else I can do," I imagine their minds protesting. I did the best I could to convey that their expressions of care and concern truly helped us both immeasurably. But Americans are an action-oriented people. This became abundantly clear as countless offers came pouring in. The generous gestures were very much appreciated. But trying to envision what "help" looked like left me feeling uncomfortable. The discomfort arose out of what I perceived as a suggestion that we let go of the reins of our life. From young ages, both Jim and I had been fiercely independent. Receiving "help" felt destabilizing. Control over our lives had already been wrestled out of our hands by cancer. My home was the last area I had dominion over. Anyone coming in to assume my domestic duties felt like a hostile takeover.

A conundrum emerged when certain offers progressed from appropriately supportive to aggressively maniacal. The one-way conversation would go something like this: "How can I help? What can I do? Do you need food? Can I clean your house? Watch the cats? Let me wash your windows!!" The words came at me like machine gun fire. I literally felt like I was being grabbed by the lapels and shaken. A bizarre verbal wrestling match would ensue. It felt like the person making the offer was trying to force me into a submissive position of victimhood that would match the model of trauma they had in their minds. At stake was my agency and sense of empowerment, so I wrestled back with polite fortitude. With some people, my gracious "no thank you" didn't dissuade them in the slightest. In fact, it seemed to embolden them as they persisted with increasingly intrusive offers. It was exhausting, so with all the strength of a coward, I solved the problem by avoiding them.

There were a few other peculiar situations. Like the friends who called late at night after they'd had a few and wanted to chat. Sigh. *Fuck sake. Go to bed,* I'd think. Or the folks who insisted on visiting and others who called daily. During these uncomfortable moments, it seemed like they were putting their needs first—a very human thing to do. Hell, I do it all the time. I cared about our friends whose emotional duress seemed to manifest in action items, but I didn't have the capacity to support them. All I could do was avoid them and hope they figured out a healthy way to sort themselves out.

I'm not upset by these awkward situations and hope people don't feel badly about my telling of them. With the growing concern about the pandemic, everyone was navigating the stress and anxiety of uncharted territory. I will be forever humbled by, and grateful for, everyone's support and love, no matter how it was expressed. In the future, maybe CaringBridge would consider setting up a group chat for people to share their feelings about a loved one's illness. That could be a useful tool for people to use as a way of getting their feelings out while diffusing the pressure felt by the patient's caregivers.

Visiting time was at a premium, which made scheduling visitors tricky. One person actually showed up unannounced during our preliminary crisis/chaos phase. The "drop-in" was presumptuous and felt incredibly intrusive. I abruptly escorted the person out. Though the incident was upsetting to everyone involved, it made me realize that I needed to quickly set parameters to accommodate Jim's need for uplifting social contact while ensuring his health wasn't compromised. There was no shortage of people who wanted to see Jim as news of his condition spread. His mom and our immediate family members got priority seating. From there it was a constant juggle—work colleagues, bandmates, neighbors, lifelong friends—the outpouring was touching. Having company cheered Jim up and made him feel "normal," but the treatments left him feeling fatigued, so any extra social interaction was downright exhausting. Jim would never send anyone away. It was up to me to communicate the rules and set boundaries. That included being vigilant about small details like people getting their flu shots before they came in. Can you imagine? Oh, for the days when flu shots were our only worry! Right before Covid, there was only one conspiracy theorist in our circle who refused a flu shot, despite the fact that it meant he couldn't spend time in person with Jim, and that was his brother Michael. I wondered if the pain of seeing Jim so sick was too great for him to bear, so he hid behind his anti-vax beliefs to avoid him. Jim didn't let on that his brother's absence hurt his feelings. He settled for phone conversations with Michael and left the spouting of righteous indignation up to me.

We declined offers from his musician friends who wanted to bring in their instruments to pick while they visited, or stage mini "get well Jim" concerts on the parking garage roof because it was emotionally difficult to tolerate. Neuropathy, one of the side effects Jim experienced, caused tingling sensations in his extremities, making it difficult for him to play. To watch his friends perform without him would have been a painful view into what his post-cancer life might look like.

There were people Jim hadn't talked to in a while who either called an inordinate number of times or practically demanded to see him. I refer to those folks as the death vultures. Their sense of urgency in the early days was unsettling. I got the feeling they wanted to "get one last visit in" before Jim died. But we weren't yet admitting defeat, so that really bugged me. Maybe they felt guilty for not having connected over time, I don't know. Whatever the reasons, the pressure was off-putting.

One person in particular was pretty persistent. Every time we scheduled a visit with him, we ended up having to cancel because, well, cancer. The gentleman was becoming increasingly frustrated with me. Finally, in the early days of Covid, he called us from the airport. He said he had just gotten back from a job in Tijuana and wanted to stop in to see Jim on his way home. Uh, no.

In fairness, other people couldn't really know the physical and psychological complexities we were grappling with. I remember when I was a young professional, one of my mentors was dying of cancer. I wanted to see her, but she wasn't accepting visitors. I remember feeling hurt by that and wondered if I'd done something wrong. We don't know any better until we do. I'm not trying to cast judgment here, or make people feel bad for their way of expressing care for Jim. I just offer what I've learned to maybe help folks in the future.

As the saying goes, "We begin to die from the moment we are born." I take those words as an invitation to recognize that the time is always right to express what's in my heart and on my mind to the people I care about. Emotional honesty is probably the greatest gift you can give to yourself and others. And I don't mean the standard "I love you man!" I mean honesty about everything from love and friendship to hurt feelings and sadness. Be real and express yourself in the moments you have together. Foster tenderness, if only for a moment. If you can do that, you'll know that while on this earth, you shared genuine human connection with people, and you won't feel like you have to rush to the side of a fallen comrade, because they will already have everything they need from you and you from them. I hope that helps.

Our sons

Often, one or both of our sons were around to overlap my trips home, so Jim rarely spent time in the hospital alone. Out of everyone, the boys were likely the most shocked at the state of affairs. Spending time with their dad helped them feel useful in the midst of an inexplicable situation.

Jim worked hard at his relationship with our sons. He was a present and caring father, though it didn't always come across that way. Throughout their formative years, Jim was firm with them. He set clear boundaries for their behavior, shared his values around family and personal responsibility, and modeled what it meant to be a good citizen in our community. Like many men, Jim wasn't taught as a child to *discuss* these expectations with the kids. Chores were mandatory. If the kids staged a resistance, their defiance was met with lots of shouting. Unlike the old days when children responded dutifully to full-throated authority, our kids shouted right back. There weren't any fragile flowers in our house.

Outside our home, Jim chaperoned countless school field trips and participated in the seemingly unending school projects. He brought the boys with him anywhere they were willing to go. Saturdays were packed with shopping trips to the Rochester Public Market, household chores and a stop at his cousin's hardware store to pick up supplies for the latest home improvement project. When the work around our house was done, Jim would take the boys to his parents' house to mow the lawn and take care of odd jobs.

Throughout their teenage years, Jim respected their need for space while trying to find ways of engaging with them. As the boys matured, their father-son relationship transitioned from one heavily laden with top-down behavior management to one marked by mutual appreciation and collaboration. They were increasingly able to enjoy each other as people, free from the old-school authoritarian power imbalance. Though less frequent, they continued to take trips together, expanding their horizons to further flung locales. Their last big adventure was a trip through Italy. A gift chockablock full of invaluable memories.

They all shared an exceptional talent for visual arts. Watching them draw together in Jim's hospital room lifted my heart with pride. The boys would show Jim their work and they'd talk together about technique and style. A lifelong learner, Jim not only enjoyed teaching the boys, but he loved learning about the latest tools, styles and techniques the kids were picking up at school. The few times I saw Jim cry during his illness occurred when he was talking about our sons. The thought of leaving them was crushing.

Jim went in the hospital before the boys' spring semesters at college started, so they were able to keep the home fires burning. Unfortunately, Gianni was present to hear Jim's diagnosis from Dr. B the day before he had to drive back to school. I imagined the news filling up his car like exhaust fumes. He wasn't having a good college experience to begin with. Facing that cold desolate road back to his rural school in the dead of winter must've felt extra terrible.

During Gianni's first full week back at school, I received a panicked phone call from him. "Mom! When I signed up for my Microsoft Office account last semester, I registered with the username 'Barry McCockiner!' I didn't need the account for my classes first semester. But this semester I have to turn in writing assignments and each one has 'Barry McCockiner' stamped at the top! I'M GONNA GET EXPELLED!" He didn't think anyone else could see his sign-in name when he made the account and he couldn't figure out how to change it.

Gianni has what I politely refer to as an "edgy" sense of humor. It takes a lot for me to be shocked by his words. My parental context combined with the fact that my brain was 98% preoccupied meant I didn't get the problem right away. I thought it was merely a sophomoric attempt at humor because the name had the word "cock" in it, so I was dismissive. I told him that it would be fine and he should suck it up and call the IT folks. He insisted that he couldn't call the IT people because "in this climate" he would most definitely get expelled. About 12 hours later, I said the name out loud to myself. That's when it dawned on me. I got a hearty laugh out of how slow I was on the uptake. Then Jim and I laughed even harder at our son.

As for our Rochester college student, he literally was spreading himself—and his possessions—between his apartment and our house. When I came home one day for my daily ablutions, Giacomo had left his "peace pipe" on the coffee table, along with the legal-ish contents. He was slowly turning our living room into his bedroom. Bleh. I hate that. Our home was becoming a wild frontier. His time was occupied with school and with work so the cats weren't getting the attention they were used to. Man, it doesn't take long for animals (and young men) to go all feral. I had to call in reinforcements to establish some semblance of order. Obviously, he was grown, so I couldn't hire a babysitter. But I had something better in mind. Grammy. My mother was very eager to help in any way she could, but at 84 years old, she struggled with multiple ailments that prevented her from tackling any of the domestic tasks like cleaning or cooking. Still, in her mind, she was 45 and could do anything she wanted to. That's a dangerous combination. Denial runs strong in that one. Though she wasn't physically able to help out, her mere presence provided a distraction. Ever respectful and loving of his grandmother, my son had to clean up and be on his best behavior. It was a mutually beneficial situation where they both took care of each other—not in the way they believed they were, but it worked out all the same.

I don't know what was going through our sons' minds as they spent every free minute they could muster with their father. Would they view those days as a gift of time to be cherished? Or a painful curse? Love and suffering were interwoven so tightly, I marvel at their bravery to sit with their feelings.

The family area

The family waiting area was pleasant and comfortable enough for visits that were relatively short. The space looked like a fat hallway with tables and chairs. Some of the chairs were cushioned two-seaters, but you wouldn't characterize them as couches. The carpet-less floor established a cold, institutional feeling that couldn't be erased by the modest comforts provided.

One side of the hall was adorned with a bank of floor to ceiling windows that created an illusion of space. When shining, the sun filled the hall with its dazzling brilliance. Depending on the weather, you could see the Wendy's across the street or as far away as the rolling landscapes of Bristol to the south of the city. The beautiful view sometimes helped us forget that we were in such an anxious and stressful place. At the end of the bank of windows, there was a small corner with children's toys and a galley kitchen equipped with coffee service, a microwave and a "Patients Only" refrigerator.

A number of colorful jigsaw puzzles in various stages of completion decorated the tables. Puzzle solving was a communal effort, providing comfort to those in waiting. It seemed like the one thing we had control over, where we could observe progress and rejoice in our collective creation. A completed puzzle was proudly displayed for several days before it was returned to its box. Sometimes, if I couldn't sleep, I'd wander down the corridor to add some pieces to someone's work in progress. Puzzle assembly invited a welcome meditative activity at 2 a.m. Though all alone, I felt supported by the previous participants. The silent, autonomous collective emitted a vibe of caring solidarity that lingered in the room long after people were gone.

An entire family was camped out there during our first full week in the center. I believe they were waiting for their person to pass. They tried their best to sleep on the chairs. It looked terribly uncomfortable. I thought it was beautiful that despite the uninviting accommodations, so many of the family members wanted to be together in the gloaming of their loved one's life.

The family area was a strange juxtaposition of those preparing for death next to people who were actively working on living. The intermingling reminded me of the Saguenay River in Quebec. For Jim's 40th birthday, I surprised him with a trip to Quebec City. As part of our vacation, I booked a whale-watching trip on the Saguenay River. The saltwater from the St. Lawrence Estuary (one of the largest and deepest estuaries on the planet) blends into the fresh water of the Saguenay, creating an amazing combination of flora and fauna. It's a perfect feeding ground for Beluga and Minke whales. You can actually whale-watch as far inland as the Saguenay Fjord.

This fat hallway was like an estuary, setting the stage for life's tug-of-war to play out with patients and doctors on one side and the natural course of life on the other. It was populated by people in various states of determination, grief, fear, joy, sadness, and resignation. We saw people living fiercely, holding death off for as long as they could while others quietly relented, giving in to eternal slumber. The ecosystem supported a confluence of family members on an emotional spectrum. At any given moment, you'd find some people praying for miracles, while others were praying for death. Many were seeking comfort while grappling with realism. It's as uncommon an ecosystem as the Saguenay. I was waiting for a whale to come in and start working on a puzzle.

Despite the brackish undercurrent, peoples' spirits injected a good vibe. The pandemic had yet to scorch the earth, so the area was highly trafficked with visitors. It was in this makeshift living room that Jim would receive guests. It felt dignified, like we were entertaining company rather than getting a visit because he was sick. Jim was a very social man. He loved having people over. Before kids and big jobs, we used to host random acts of visitors at our home all the time. My brother once likened our porch to a coffee shop.

The change of scenery was welcome. We'd go there to hang out sometimes to get away from the monitors. The first time we sat there together, Jim looked up at the artwork on the wall and exclaimed: "I know that place! That's Jason's land!" He took a picture of the painting and sent it to his friend Jason right then and there to verify. Sure enough, one of their mutual artist friends had spent time on Jason's land in Bristol, painting. The scene was of Jason's pond. Jim hunted the land with Jason many times over the years. When the boys were young, Jim would take them up there to mess around and canoe on that very pond.

Jim had so many fond memories attached to Jason's place. One early summer day when the kids were little, Jim took the boys and our German Shepard Roxanne there to fish. They got in the canoe and rowed out to the middle of the pond. Unbeknownst to them, a family of snakes had made their home in the bottom of the canoe. The activity woke them up and they started slithering around. Gianni thought it was the neatest thing he ever saw. Giacomo, on the other hand, flipped his shit. Jim was trying to balance the canoe as the boys hopped up and down: one out of joyful excitement and the other out of terror. Roxanne, who had been left on shore, swam out to them and tried to get in the boat to find out what all the excitement was about. Total mayhem. The transcendent presence of that painting provided a deep comfort to Jim's soul.

Receiving guests in the family area not only helped us maintain some sense of normalcy, but it kept everyone out of our most personal business inside Jim's actual room. Jim had so many different physical issues resulting from the chemotherapy. It was embarrassing enough to have to go through all of that in front of strangers. Receiving visitors in his room felt intrusive. The room was like our cocoon. Our family was sharing an intimacy that would not be easily replicated under any other circumstance, and we couldn't bear to extend it beyond us four.

As I met more people at the coffee maker, I realized how fortunate we were to live so close to the hospital. I could literally run to the cancer center from our house in 20 minutes. We weren't the norm. So many families were traveling miles and miles to get there. One morning, I met a woman who lived over an hour away. She was trying to be present for her husband while cobbling together people to manage her house and care for her pets. She would have to leave to go home and bridge the gaps. I can't imagine what her drives were like. The agony of leaving her husband, worrying about him while home, and then the ensuing anxiety over what she'd find while driving toward him. The adrenalin and cortisol flowing through her veins must have wreaked havoc on her body. And she wasn't a young woman. Once, her husband was discharged only to return the very next day because he was experiencing complications. What sheer hell.

CHAPTER TEN

The "Lay" of the Land

Jim had an amazing body. There were plenty of nicknames bandied about by friends and family that acknowledged this fact. The band community called him "Jimmy Guns." I've heard "Fabio" tossed around over the years and our eldest referred to him as "Tarzan." Jim worked out regularly ever since he was in the military some 38 years ago. But he wasn't a gym rat. My husband was a "do-it-yourselfer" in all aspects of his life, including fitness. He was a regular runner and observed a daily calisthenics regimen. He was in the habit of doing sit-ups, push-ups and pull-ups almost every single day, wherever he was. Our neighbors have fond memories of seeing him in the schoolyard across the street doing pull-ups and sit-ups on the playground. The only fitness gear he would spend money on was his sneakers. And even then, he'd run them into the ground before he'd buy new ones. In the summer, he ran in his swim trunks and rarely wore a shirt, completing his Tarzan-like appearance. I'll never forget the summer he decided to wear a do-rag to keep the sweat out of his eyes and his hair out of his face. Did I mention Jim was gifted with a significant proboscis? Oh my God! I got the biggest kick out of that whole scene. I told him he looked like a nose in sneakers.

Jim was of average height, about five-foot-eleven. Kyphosis caused a curve in his spine that became a noticeable hunch in his back as he aged. Though he took great care to keep his back strong, the condition probably knocked an inch off his height by the time he got sick. I think his gregarious personality made him seem taller than he was. He had a great big barrel chest and a mile-wide smile that came quick to his lips. He would greet people with that smile and huge bear hugs. Folded in his arms, the warmth of his friendship could be felt to your marrow. I like to close my eyes and remember our tender embraces. Our hugs were spontaneous, like punctuations throughout the long sentence of our day. Feeling our hearts beat together in our embrace was meditative. The world around us disappeared while our bodies and spirits joined in a moment of pure peace and love.

I'm bereft without his body. There is no way my imagination can adequately recreate the physical feeling of his warmth or fill the vacancy in my heart left by his loss. Perhaps when my body dies, my spirit will link up with his again and restore the greatness of our love somewhere in the ether. But I'm more inclined to believe that what we had was a gift that the universe makes available maybe in consolation for some of the crappier stuff we have to deal with in life. Sometimes I wonder if the high-test love generated by two souls is just a glimpse of what the afterlife has in store for us. As I return my thoughts to the corporeal, my arrythmia that developed after Jim passed away is a constant reminder that my heart is irreparably broken.

Discovering the mini gym on his hospital floor sparked Jim's enthusiasm. In those early days, he met a couple of other patients in the gym. Chatting with them gave him that community feel he cherished so much in his life outside of cancer. And observing a fitness routine, albeit modified, restored a sense of normalcy to his day. The small room was equipped with a treadmill, stationary bike, and stairs. He'd only been in the hospital for two weeks, so he was both surprised and bummed when he got a charley horse on his first attempt to climb the stairs. Undeterred, he hopped on the stationary bike and settled into a new way of working out.

Building certain familiar activities into the day, like using the gym and walking the hospital neighborhood, gave Jim some control over his body and his schedule. He had mini goals that he could achieve. His body may not have been as strong as it was walking into the hospital, but he was driven to stave off the effects of both the cancer and the treatments. Those mini goals turned into a sense of purpose that helped his psyche cope with his situation. Through his inner strength, tenacity and determination, Jim proved that being Tarzan was more about spirit than it was about physique.

An added bonus to our cancer carnival was the major construction project going on. Yes, the hospital was so dedicated to providing Jim with a patient-centered experience that they made sure to include the nine-to-five noise of a construction site directly beneath his room—free of charge. Nail gun pops, the rumbling and hissing of air compressors, and random acts of jackhammery added an extra layer of unnerving disquiet to our environment. Jim rarely enjoyed uninterrupted sleep at night. Periodic vitals checks, medication administrations, and plain old having cancer made it difficult for Jim to enjoy the deliciousness of a deep slumber. A hospital is no place to go for rest. He was exhausted during the day, but every time he dozed off, the power tools would start up again. It's almost as if the workmen knew how to time their noise for maximum patient disturbance. We'd all have to shout at each other when the doctors and nurses came in. Trying to talk to our elderly hard-of-hearing parents on the phone was futile, so we'd cut the conversations short. It was either a sick taunt or completely obtuse when the doctors would punctuate every conversation with: "Get some rest!" Funny. I'd like to remind people that sleep deprivation is a form of torture used on prisoners since the Inquisition.

Sleep wasn't the only enjoyable activity deterred by constant interruptions. Physical intimacy was difficult to foster. Jim and I had a healthy sex life. I know the adjective "healthy" doesn't exactly evoke excitement when describing sex. I imagine you're stuck with images of Rob and Laura Petrie instead of 50 shades of hubba-hubba—the latter being what many would prefer to hear about.

So what does healthy mean? To me, healthy means we enjoyed our sex life together and made sure we tended to our physical needs on a regular basis. I wouldn't characterize it as wild in any way. We didn't swing from chandeliers or break any records. As a middle-aged couple of 30 years, we were pretty routine, focusing on personal best. But I always loved it and thought after the act "Why don't we do this more often?" In fact, that would be my only critique—one I believe my husband would agree with—more would have been great. But that was on us.

For those of you who don't know, in order for two people to have intercourse they need to be in the same room. At the same time. For us, we needed a third component: same room, same time and *relaxed*. That third component was the tricky one, because if Jim and I were in the same room, at the same time and relaxed there was an unspoken race between engaging in sex and zzzzzzzzzzz.

Overall, we managed to do pretty well and keep each other satisfied. In the hospital, after the dust settled from the first week of crisis, we sought comfort in each other's arms—the one place where we could truly console each other and provide much needed emotional care. But the environment wasn't intended to foster intimacy. Jim's room was a 24/7 revolving door of people. We never knew when anyone was going to come in. Add to the stream of people the unnerving racket emanating from the construction project below us. We definitely were not going to achieve the third component of our lovemaking formula.

Out of desperation, we retreated to the bathroom to give it a go. The bathroom was fairly large, so there was room enough. But the interior looked like Chernobyl with all the cautionary signs wallpapering the place shouting "Hazardous Material! Bathroom exclusively for patient use!" Bathroom sex didn't exactly provide the emotional comfort care we were looking for, but it was fun and checked off a bunch of other important boxes. I remember the odd look on our oncologist's face when we divulged our activity. It was a combination of horror, pity and 'good for you!' She quickly drew our attention to the section of the new cancer patient information packet that discussed necessary precautions around engaging in intercourse with someone receiving chemotherapy. From there on out, we made sure to plan our lovemaking around treatments to protect me from getting poisoned by the stuff. I'm surprised I didn't glow in the dark after our first liaison.

CHAPTER ELEVEN

Treatment

Due to the fact that Jim burst onto the hospital scene in a spectacularly critical condition, he was sentenced to inpatient chemo treatments. The doctors had to monitor his progress closely to track how he was tolerating the assault. Chemo poisons kill all rapidly growing cells—good and bad—wiping out everything in their path like Sullivan's Campaign. Hospitalization allowed for ease of intervention if Jim's body chemistry went out of whack in response to the treatments. Kidney and liver function, the mass in his chest, platelets, electrolytes—there were so many things to keep track of. He was already starting from a position of weakness because of the lymphoblast pool party in his mediastinum. Immunosuppression was another result of the beatdown. Our hypervigilance around cleanliness and minimizing Jim's exposure to folks became good practice for the looming Covid pandemic.

The treatments were administered in phases, and each phase had a cycle. Jim's first phase was called the "induction" phase. The process began with the oncologist writing orders for a specific poison cocktail. In this case, it was Daunorubicin and

Vincristine. We called it Donna Robinson and Vinnie Cristina because it was easier to remember and we could blame those two jerks for making Jim feel crappy. Jim had already started on the Dexamethasone steroid a couple days earlier. The chemo prescription would get sent to a special part of the hospital pharmacy for filling. We envisioned a dim, dusty lab with hunchbacks, cauldrons, witches, and maniacal Mr. Hyde-like dudes toiling away over the noxious concoctions.

Everything had to be timed properly because the chemo medication expired relatively quickly, I guess. Or ate through the container it was in, I'm not sure which. When the poison was ready, two nurses dressed in hazmat suits would bring in the bags of chemicals, hang them on the IV pole and connect them to Jim's PICC line. The process kind of reminded me of pumping gas in a car. The nurses carefully checked each other through every step of the process. It was remarkable how efficiently and expertly the nurses worked together. If this was what we had to go through to fight cancer, at least the agents of delivery were good at what they were doing. The nurses would let him be while the noxious chemicals dripped into his veins. Once the poison was administered, they'd unhook him and from there on out, we'd all manage the side effects together.

Children who have this disease get blasted with higher doses of chemo, referred to as the "Pediatric Protocol." Though it sounds horrible, it makes sense because kids are little cell growth factories. Still, seeing how the doses affected Jim, it broke my heart to think that little kids are subjected to an even more rigorous regimen.

The oncology nurses, individually and as a collective, were outstanding. They were kind and compassionate masters of their profession. As we talked with them, we learned that many were driven to work in the cancer center because of their own personal experiences with the disease. Their empathy was genuine. Over the course of our stay, many spent time chatting with Jim. The subjects covered a wide range of topics—Italy, Rochester, art and music. He was always interested in other people's family origins and how they became nurses in the cancer center. Jim was a talker and he found plenty of willing conversationalists in the nursing staff.

We can't escape the fact that Death is always walking with us. The halls of the cancer center are a prime spot for the Grim Reaper to rack up steps. The nurses were well aware of the dark shadow that lingered around every corner. Their ability to respectfully coexist with Death added a divinity to their nature. They did everything they could to help Jim thwart the advancing Reaper, and when everyone's best efforts didn't manifest the outcome we wanted, they remained steadfast, compassionate and emotionally available. They bore witness to the awesome power and great mystery of life.

The rounding team was made up of doctors in various stages of credentialing, nurse practitioners, and nurse managers. They would come in every morning any time between nine and noon-ish. This was when we felt most like zoo animals on display. To reiterate, the rounding team was a bunch of strangers led by a resident and an attending physician, who came in to check on my half-naked husband. The resident was our dedicated physician for the duration of their rotation. This doctor in training wasn't necessarily interested in becoming an oncologist. "Rotating" through the different departments was a requirement of their training. Their role was to keep an eye on Jim and to provide any necessary medical interventions to stabilize him during chemo treatments.

The resident opened the session by presenting a summary of Jim's health status to the attending while the others stood and stared at us. After the brief update, the resident would double-check with Jim to make sure they were on the same page with him and that they hadn't left anything out. The attending spoke next. He or she would ask Jim questions about how he was feeling and about his bodily functions. What was particularly infantilizing was the focus on Jim's bowel movements and urine output. Every time he peed, he had to use a handheld urinal and save it for the nurses to measure. Jim's urinary evacuation performance was a key indicator of his kidney function and other internal workings, measured because there's an awful domino effect of adverse issues if one little thing goes wrong.

We understood the necessity, but the knowledge didn't make the hyper-attention any less embarrassing. Everyone was good natured about this personal invasion, but it's dehumanizing to have to engage in these conversations with a group of strangers, some of whom are half your age, while barely dressed. Seriously, one morning, when you're barely awake, try to imagine 10 people piling into your bedroom, pulling off your blankets and scrutinizing your body.

Once the two doctors were done asking questions, they checked his vitals, paying particular attention to his heart and lungs. Occasionally one of the other people in the group would add information to our sessions, but most of the time, they observed quietly. The meeting would end with a Q & A from us. They'd do their best to answer our questions.

We sidestepped the big question that was top of mind: Will Jim survive? As you might imagine, that's as hard a question to answer as it is to ask. We feared the question would open the door to a bumbling collection of words that would feature discomfort and ambiguity as our audience tried to marry science with hope, so we avoided asking. But it nagged at me every day, if not every five minutes.

Rather than suffer that exchange, we saved our prognosis and treatment plan questions for our team captain, Dr. B. We'd have to wait to connect with her because she worked full time in the outpatient center. Which meant we had to catch her before her day started or find her on breaks between her other patients and responsibilities. The communication gap between us was exacerbated by life events. When we got back from the ICU, she was out sick for a week, then took a week vacation. It was tough because she was the only doctor I really wanted to talk to.

The residents assigned to Jim clearly wanted to do a good job, but despite their good nature and commitment, it was hard to feel confident in their ability to take care of Jim. They weren't oncologists, and their experience was minimal. They were winging it, fresh out of school. The cancer center doctors all knew Jim had a bad disease, and they must have suspected his time was limited. Why then wouldn't they have reconfigured his treating team to rely more on experienced doctors and less on residents? (Pausing here to let you ponder the cost savings likely involved with the student staffing decision.) Including the phrase "patient-centered care" multiple times in informational materials they give you upon hospital admission doesn't manifest that experience. Actions speak louder than words—and those actions were telling us that our hospital's priority was the education and training of their residents.

Jim, as a patient, was docile, which is not a characteristic anyone would have thought to assign to my husband. He had a lot of energy and enthusiasm for life. Jim was passionate about his multiple endeavors, and he didn't shy away from disagreements (that's a polite way of saying he could be a strident, argumentative S.O.B.). I found it disconcerting when his forthright, live-out-loud personality settled into one of quiet acquiescence.

Without fail, when the doctors came in on rounds and asked him how he was, he'd reply in a chipper voice: "I'm fine. How are you?" rather than "I have a fucking shitty cancer! I feel sick all the time! I can't crap! My body hurts! I hate feeling nauseous and dopey! This bed is shit! I hate your TV! I'm terrified of dying! I don't want to leave my family! I have no idea if any of this crap is going to save my life, and it just plain sucks!"

I mean, he didn't have to go that far, but somewhere in between "everything's fine" and "everything is shit" would have provided a more accurate picture for the doctors. As his advocate, this situation plagued me throughout his care. When something was bothering him, I'd call the doctors and nurses who would come in at my behest, only to be told by Jim that everything was "ok." He'd play his symptoms down like they were no big thing. Argh! It was so frustrating! Often, he would do this while I wasn't in the room. I'd only find out later when I thought no one was following up. The nurses would tell me "We already talked to him about it, and he said he was okay." This led to one of the few arguments we had in the hospital. Exasperated, I told him "I look like a crazy person! You aren't gonna get the care you need if you keep telling everyone everything is fine!"

Jim and I communicated volumes without words. That's not to say we didn't talk—no one could accuse either of us of being short on words—it's just that when you've been in a close relationship with someone for so long you share more silently than you realize. Kind of like how trees communicate to each other through their root systems. Our marital telepathy let me know for example that the attention Jim received from the rounding doctors made him incredibly uncomfortable. He was a humble man who never liked being the center of attention. Based on his love of performance, one would not infer that this was the case. But when you perform in a band, you're enjoying a shared experience while your audience appreciates the ensemble as a whole, not just you. In this situation, the intense attention embarrassed him. He felt like he was a bother to all these professional people, so he downplayed his symptoms when he responded to the doctor's questions. He was reluctant to accept the fact that he *was* their work and *the reason* they were all there. I also knew that he was scared and felt powerless over his disease. He was sincere when he asked the doctors how *they* were—it was his way of normalizing their interactions to dilute his fear.

When the doctors asked him the battery of questions during rounds, I needed to gently coax him past the polite, self-effacing responses and into honest answers about his condition. I stood by and listened as the conversation ran its appropriate course. It was his body, his cancer. He had been stripped of all control. I had no interest in adding to his feeling of disempowerment by interrupting or correcting him. But what Jim was relating to the doctors and what he was actually experiencing often were two different things. Between his fear and the opioids, clarity wasn't always the point of order. The doctors knew I was there all the time, so they would look at me while they talked with Jim to see if my body language was supporting what Jim was saying. I appreciated that tacit understanding. Unfortunately, though, there were times I could feel a bias *against* me from some of the professionals who were new to us. Maybe they had come across one too many women who were fluent in "womansplain," or had suffered the aggression of domineering spouses who spoke for their partners.

Don't get me wrong, over 30 years I made my share of mistakes in this area. I'm no sinless princess here. However, as I mentioned earlier, Jim and I learned a lot together over the years about how to see and hear each other. Working through all our relationship issues over the years prepared me for these complex communications. When Jim was finished answering the questions, it was my turn to tell the doctors what I knew to be true. Like the resident would look to me for confirmation, I looked at Jim while I talked, checking in with him to make sure I was getting it right.

We were simultaneously strong and fragile—strong as we endured the trappings of cancer and fragile in our fears about losing our lives to an invisible foe. Jim *wanted* everything to be fine. He *wanted* the doctors to be people he met in the bar—people he was just having a chat with. He could not stand the fact that he was sick. To some degree, I think his mind was pretending he wasn't.

CHAPTER TWELVE

February

Two weeks and three chemo treatments later, things were looking up. The original complications caused by the disease were under control. The chemo treatments seemed to be working. There was optimism in the air! Our oncologist granted Jim a "hall pass," allowing him to go home for the day. The care providers all knew how important home was to us. I'm not certain, but I think for insurance purposes, we could only leave for a couple hours. I got the impression that the insurance company would stop paying for inpatient care if they found out the patient was out of the hospital for some legally-determined amount of time. Despite the short timeframe, it was really great for Jim to be home, sitting on our couch and petting the cats. He actually *wanted* to do the dishes! Watching him engage in this household chore made me realize how important routine tasks are to the infrastructure of our identities. Being home together turned our anxiety dial way down for a few short hours. Unbeknownst to us at the time, it was a reprieve before the next storm hit.

Our hearts were set on achieving outpatient status the following week, which would get Jim home in time for

Valentine's Day. Valentine's Day was never a high priority occasion for us, but this year, it seemed like a nice date to mark Jim's return home. On February 11th, with hope in my heart, I started packing the few creature comforts I had brought to Jim's room, in order to get ahead of what we thought was our impending discharge. I decided to sleep at home that evening to get a full night's rest in anticipation of Jim's move home. The nights I wasn't in the hospital, I left strict instructions for the staff to call me if anything happened, so I was relatively comfortable allowing myself the luxury of a good night's sleep.

That night, Jim was struck with excruciating pain in his ribs. Though it was cause for concern among the night team, no one contacted me. That morning, none the wiser, I called Jim before I left the house to see how his night was and if he needed me to bring anything in particular before I came back. That's when I found out he was in pain. There wasn't enough room in my worried mind to be furious with the night crew. I moved so fast, I'm not even sure how I got to the hospital. When I walked into his room, I found him crumpled up on his bed in the fetal position. The night crew ran several tests on him to rule out a repeat of the issues that landed him in the ICU. While doing so, they tried a couple of medicines to mitigate the pain. Ironically, they started with Tylenol, which is like bringing a butter knife to a gun fight. Thank goodness someone had the presence of mind to kick it up a few notches with a stronger pain medicine. Still, whatever they were giving him wasn't providing any relief, so by the time I got there, he was in agony.

Later that morning the doctors figured out that the cancer indeed was fighting back. The chemo wasn't working. The news sucked the air out of our lungs. They started a pain management regimen and gave him more of the steroid inflammation fighter, Dexamethasone, to give him some relief. Dr. B instructed the team to continue with the current chemo regimen as planned while she researched a stronger chemo recipe. They had to keep using the fire hose they had until they could arrange for a water cannon.

This was a crushing setback. And we really didn't know what to make of it. We were saturating our piped-in hospital air with the trepidation steaming off of our bodies. By the end of the week, we were desperate to hear that *something* was going to work. Rather than waiting to talk to Dr. B, we met our attending physician on rounds with all our ramped-up fear and asked her the question we had been avoiding: What happened if the new chemo regimen didn't work? She looked us dead in the eyes and said there was nothing more they could do.

Now, I've likely mentioned ad nauseum that I'm a practical person. I want to know what I'm dealing with so we can plan accordingly. However, this doctor was way out of line for dropping that on us without any support—from our oncologist, from a therapist or social worker—*anybody* who had the human sense to have a longer, appropriate conversation with us about prognosis and options. It was like her fucked up mic drop moment. She matter-of-factly, in the middle of rounds, while we were completely unprepared, told us, "There are no other options." There's another one who needed a good hard slap. How can these professionals be so stupid?

When we finally got to talk to Dr. B, we told her what the attending said. She was disturbed and asked out loud "Why would she tell you that?" Of course, Jim and I couldn't answer that question. Then she assured us that there were other options if this next chemo recipe didn't work. I can't say we were awash with relief. We came away from that conversation with something south of cautious optimism.

While Dr. B worked on a new concoction, the rest of us spent the week managing Jim's pain and waiting for him to take a crap. For the pain, they started Jim on an oral form of the narcotic, Dilaudid. That didn't do much, so they escalated the Dilaudid to an IV drip. The hospital used a 1–10 pain scale, to calibrate the dosing that would bring Jim some relief: one represented the least amount of pain and 10 the highest. I estimated for example that the morning I found him in the fetal position, he was at a 10.

Jim's self-dismissing behavior became a big barrier to narrowing in on the course of action. This was one of the most frustrating experiences of my married life. He would tell me he was in pain—not words my husband was given to use. Then, the doctor would come in and ask the "1–10" pain scale question. Jim would rate his pain at a three or four. "Three or four" doesn't typically require opioids. Jim was definitely in greater pain, but for some reason, he wouldn't use a higher number. Was it a generation thing? Would a 23-year-old man say he was at a nine to Jim's three? A circular problem started where the resident would prescribe pain medications based on Jim's low-ball number. Then he'd get behind the pain, meaning his pain was greater than what he was being prescribed so it would reach an intolerable level. The resident wasn't able to manage the pain with what they were prescribing, so they'd have to catch up with more pain medication to wrestle it under control before they could settle down to a consistent pain management regimen. If you can't control the pain, other parts of the body get affected. Your heart rate goes up and other systems in your body get stressed. It's a delicate equilibrium that requires close attention. The attempts to get the medications right were an everyday, all-day frustration.

After several days of this back and forth, I scrapped the useless number scale. Somehow, I had to find a way to develop a shared definition for pain levels that accurately described Jim's pain so everyone had a clear understanding of where we were. I ended up making a picture chart to replace the hospital's number scale. Each picture had a pain description using words I heard Jim use over the course of the week. Then I added numbers for the team. As an artist, Jim communicated best through pictures. The most important picture was my depiction of Jim doubled over like he was the night the cancer was fighting back. I gave that picture a nine knowing Jim would never admit to a 10 in any circumstance.

The break in the clouds came when a new nurse came on rotation. She pulled me aside and promptly threw the resident under the bus. She said that Jim needed to be seen by the palliative care team and that the current care providers shouldn't be yo-yoing Jim, trying to guess at right medicines, timing, and dosing. Initially, fear struck my heart when she said "palliative" because I thought palliative care was specifically for people who were dying. She explained that the palliative team specialized in pain management and that they can be brought in to collaborate for anyone's care. She said she was going to tell the resident, but wanted me to know first. Relieved, I thanked her and supported her direction.

I got the impression that this disclosure on her part served a dual purpose. She genuinely wanted to include me in her thought process that would likely help Jim, *and* she wanted me to know that she knew better than the resident. I certainly appreciated her insight and recommendation. I didn't think her approach—criticizing the resident to a patient—was very professional. Yet *another* indicator of a haphazard hospital culture. Despite the overarching institutional problems, the nurse's intervention resulted in better care for Jim. As with all these issues, I continued to press on, saving my "patient experience" reflections for another day.

In hindsight, this situation highlights the fact that our experience was student-focused. And, it makes me realize that while we were in the hospital, we didn't have a coach at all. We had an oncologist writing the strategy, but that physician wasn't part of the day-to-day. There wasn't any one present person overseeing what was happening to us. That's why a nurse had to step in and lead from behind.

As cancer patients know, one treatment often leads to the need for another. In this instance, narcotics have a constipating effect. Constipation causes other problems, so there was intense interest in Jim's bowel movements. Valentines' week, Jim was grappling with bone pain, headaches, reflux, and constipation. The resurgence of Jim's cancer dashed all our hopes of a Valentine's Day discharge. Instead, helping Jim move his bowels became the project of the week. What a change in plans.

The team first prescribed Senna, a natural laxative. My husband's gastrointestinal system didn't even register that folderol. Next, they gave him lactulose—another laxative that proved ineffective. They moved on to a stronger evacuant called MiraLAX. That one at least got the attention of Jim's colon, but it remained stubbornly stoned. The narcotics were too enjoyable. These laxatives were like little kids bothering their father while he was napping in a hammock. "Come on Dad! Come play with us!" "Rmph." Jim was starting to barf more because of all the backup in his system. When MiraLAX didn't work, things got serious. The resident came in wearing a hazmat suit, pushing a wheelbarrow carrying a frighteningly large jug labeled with the best misnomer I've ever seen: Golytely. (BTW, JK re: hazmat suit and wheelbarrow) Golytely was miserable stuff. Jim tried to drink it, but it made him barf more. At this point, he was so full of shit, everything made him vomit. Enter stage left—fear of dehydration and damaged kidney function. Man, what a misery. Trying to simultaneously help him shit, hydrate, manage the pain and deal with all the other chemo side effects. Fuck all.

Finally, on Valentine's Day, I'd reached the end of my rope. He hadn't pooped in days and was flirting with increased complications, so I started working on him like you would a constipated toddler. I got him unhooked from his IV leash and bent him width-wise over the hospital bed—the best substitute for an exercise ball. I started "Operation Bowel Movement" by massaging his back. Once he was relaxed, I gradually increased my pressure with the heels of my hands on his lower back and flanks. I kept kneading and pressing and rolling my hands in a circular motion on his back and sides. Jim was doing his own work to move it all through internally, instructing me on what was most useful. A light at the end of the tunnel appeared (so to speak) when Jim announced that he could feel some progress, so he disrobed and got into the shower. He crouched down under the soothing warm water while I, fully clothed, continued to knead the muscles in his back. After what felt like hours of massaging, and heaving and ho'ing and yoga positioning, Jim gave birth to a massive pile of shit. Oh my God! We were so relieved! We both felt an incredible sense of accomplishment!

With what little energy he had left, Jim cleaned up and crept back into his hospital bed. Equally exhausted, I crawled in next to him and snuggled up by his side. While couples far and wide were saying "I love you" over romantic dinners, or sharing champagne and chocolates, Jim and I were expressing the truest love for each other over the delivery of a much-anticipated bowel movement.

Not only were our hopes dashed for a February 14 discharge, the latest turn of events meant we needed to stay even longer. Resigned to our disappointing reality, I retrieved the things I'd brought home, and added a few more creature comforts to the bag. As I said earlier, we didn't want the hospital to be our home, or our "new normal." But the whole situation was so depressing; I wanted to have things around that would cheer Jim up a little while I tended to his needs.

The lymphoblasts were definitely staging an offensive in response to the first wave chemo assault. To combat the resurgence, Jim's oncologist wrote a prescription for a stronger chemo regimen. This new cycle was referred to as "salvage" chemo. That's not an adjective a patient wants to hear used to describe their treatment. It's called salvage when your cancer is refractory, meaning it's not responding to the previous treatments. For Jim, this new chemo cocktail incorporated a drug called Nelarabine. Nasty stuff.

A couple days after his last treatment in the new cycle, the night nurse found Jim standing in the bathroom staring in the mirror. He didn't know how he got there. His mental state was terrifying. I'd ask him a simple question, like "What day is it today?" He'd stare off without acknowledging me. After a few minutes he'd say something like "What?" and that was it. He was in this weird, somnolent state. I started to freak out. The explanations went round robin, with one doctor blaming the opiates, while another nurse said with certitude that it was hospital delirium. The oncologist seemed very reluctant to say it was neurotoxicity from the Nelarabine, which was the answer that made the most sense to me as Jim's primary observer.

In Jim's medical records, it says his mental vacation was multifactorial. It was explained to me that if your kidneys aren't functioning well, the opiates can dam up, sitting in your system longer than normal. Coupled with neurotoxicity from the chemo and his jumbled sense of time from being in the hospital for 39 days, I can understand that the physicians would be inclined to blame all those things. But I had been with Jim the entire time. The only time he demonstrated this kind of loss of mental function came after he had a full course of Nelarabine. For reasons unbeknownst to me, the doctors were reluctant to attribute Jim's state to this chemo drug. I'd been in the hospital for 39 days as well and I was on my last nerve. I kept asking for Dr. B to come up and see for herself what was happening. She called Jim's room and said she'd come up to see him, but she never did come to witness his drug-induced dementia. I finally asked her if she was avoiding us. Of course, she said "No," but I wonder if her subconscious was driving that bus.

To make matters worse, when the doctors came in, Jim rallied and somehow was able to answer their questions. Albeit slowly, but he'd answer. It absolutely drove me out of my goddamn tree. Still, I can't believe they didn't notice the profound difference in his cognitive abilities. Or maybe they did, but didn't want to freak me out? I'm not sure. All I know is that my husband was acting like he'd had a lobotomy and no one seemed to be nearly as alarmed as I was.

I had very few public meltdowns in the hospital. This persistent lack of interest by our doctors in what was a very big deal to me was one of those moments that tipped me over the edge into expressively frantic. Exasperated with gusto, I told the attending on rounds that Jim was acting like Jack Nicholson at the end of *One Flew Over the Cuckoo's Nest*. You know what? That attending cracked a smile! He caught himself and immediately adjusted his emotionless mask, but I saw that smile and it made a world of difference to me. You may think I'm crazy, but I received his smile as a sign that he was a human being who was seeing and hearing *me* as a human being. For once, all my thoughts and feelings were being validated. I was so tired of the mind-numbing monotone voices and the robotic stares from the rounding team, day in and day out. I had to keep myself from hugging this guy for joining me in a brief moment of shared humanity.

After struggling with everything we had struggled with, I was so hoping to get Jim home that week. With this new complication, I was starting to worry that we'd never get there. In our healthcare system, it feels like there's a disconnect between treating the patient and treating the person. Picture a balance scale with one on each side. When you're in a hospital the *patient* side of the scale is weighted down by assessments, tests, and treatments. The longer the hospital stay, the weightier the patient side becomes while the *person* side of the scale shrinks. If it stays that way too long, the person starts to suffer in ways that can badly detract from the work that's being done on the patient side. Hospitalization becomes antithetical, treating the patient to death, so to speak.

Certain environmental factors that keep a person physically and mentally stabilized in regular life are simply not available while in the hospital. Basics like the comfort of your bed, the company of your pets, and cooking your own food. Being able to drive your car, and go to your closet to pick out your clothes—these seemingly small familiarities we take for granted help our brains maintain a psychological equilibrium. Moving around freely in the environment we create for ourselves is what makes us feel like a whole person and is a large part of how we define ourselves. Though the importance of these factors in the health of a patient is acknowledged repeatedly by the doctors, who want to get you home as well, their focus stays on the disease. This is another one of those conversations I imagine the medical community engages in, but can't resolve on its own, so it gets shoved in a mental drawer somewhere only to be reflected on while staring into one's coffee.

CHAPTER THIRTEEN

Home Again, Home Again, Jiggety-Jig

When we left the hospital, Jim transitioned from a health *system* to health *care*. Living in the health system was like riding in Dorothy's house through the tornado. Shades of gray muted everything as the world spun around us, hurling the contents of our lives past our window.

Our emergence into health *care* was greeted by all the colorful cheerfulness of Munchkinland. It was a welcome change that excited our senses. Jim's patient/person balance scale tipped comfortably back toward the person side. Reclaiming some control over the basics of our lives charged our optimism. The change was a marvelous relief.

Jim's care in the outpatient center felt like a loving embrace, provided by one consistent team of people led by his oncologist. I now understood that *this* was Dr. B's natural habitat and *this* was the real team experience the cancer center was offering.

Getting discharged didn't mean we were in the clear. Jim only graduated from "inpatient" to "outpatient" status. We still had to report to the Cancer Center regularly for chemotherapy and other infusions, and a nurse came to our house several times a week to check in, take blood samples, and provide any support we needed. But a semblance of normalcy was restored to our lives as we entered a new phase of our war with cancer.

Though we visited the hospital and had in-home visiting nurse support, I assumed responsibility for Jim's day-to-day care. I have a caring and compassionate disposition, but I'm not gentle or delicate. Exhibit A: If there was a graveyard for broken dishes, the section for dearly departed earthenware from the Sanfilippo-Barbero household would occupy a large mausoleum. I buy all of our dishes, glasses, and cups second hand because they are garbage-bound within months of purchase. Jim was well aware of my limitations. For years he referred to my hands as "big, Polish onion-pickin' mitts." I can hear him now: "Jesus Jennifer! Take it easy!"

Caring for Jim was a duty I assumed gladly and without hesitation. I tended to all of his needs when he was sick from chemo, managing his medicines, finding the foods and drinks he could stomach and orienting him at night for his frequent trips to the bathroom. He playfully referred to me as "Nurse Jennifer" when I squirted the contents of the saline flushes for the PICC line onto the ceiling.

As I reflect on the difference between inpatient and outpatient care, the haunting questions about timing worm their way into my brain. I'm still afraid to ask our oncologist if Jim had gone to the doctor as soon as he felt his pain, would we have avoided that crazy roller coaster of a hospital stay altogether? If we had reacted sooner, could the doctors have prevented the pool party in his chest, stopping the spread of cancer in its tracks before he became critical? Could we have enjoyed more time together at home? My mind often alights on those thoughts like a spring robin on an iceberg.

Home sweet home is one of those expressions that has become a folksy platitude. But when we returned home together on February 28, we felt the essence of the expression wash over us. There was a palpable sweetness in the air and a warm serenity cocooned us. As March rolled in, Mother Nature gifted us with an early and prolonged spring—an uncommon occurrence for Great Lakes homesteaders. We worked so hard for years to build a good life in a comfortable home. Now, we were able to coast on the fruits of our labor and turn our attentions to the carefree aspects of homemaking.

In the receding snow of winter, we planted baby lettuce in a mini-greenhouse I learned how to make from a YouTube video. Jim drove me to the store to buy the needed components: a bag of dirt and a seed pack. There was hardly anyone at the store—evidence of a looming pandemic. As I got in the car after my quick shop, we watched an older gentleman angrily kick a shopping cart. It was the strangest thing. There wasn't a soul anywhere near him. He just marched from the parking lot toward the store entrance and kicked a cart before he went in the store. That's when I knew the psychological strain of the pandemic was going to reverberate through our populace long after the virus was wrestled under control.

When we got home, we went straight out back in the snow and cold of March to pick a good spot. We followed the directions, carefully laying the bag on the ground and cutting away plastic flaps on the top, exposing the rich, brown soil. I spread the seeds all around the rectangle of dirt. We put a clear plastic tub over the mini-garden to create the greenhouse effect and caringly bundled the base in hay. We waited patiently over the next few weeks, watching for our baby lettuces to sprout.

Meanwhile, in the warmth of our dining room, I started a tomato nursery. A quarter of the room became an incubator for a beautiful array of tomato seedlings. I never had any success with these kinds of projects in the past, likely because I didn't pay the proper attention. This time, attention was the only currency I had to pay in exchange for a fun occupation that would keep my mind off the cancer.

While I played farmer, Jim took to making bread. My mom supported his endeavors virtually, sending him different recipes and links to demonstration videos for easy baking methods. There's something timeless and beautiful about sharing the process of making bread with loved ones. I can think of no other activity that better epitomizes the essence of "home." Dating as far back as 8000 BC, the art of making bread has been passed on through the generations. Over time bread has solidified its place as a culinary foundation for many cultures in some form or fashion. Making bread is an experience that delightfully engages all our senses. It also taps into the deep recesses of our brains to channel our connection to ancestral rituals, thereby providing a spiritual comfort as well. One can sense the presence of their forebearers in a sort of existential crowd-sourced collaborative as they knead dough. The two-millennia-old story of the last supper depicts Jesus symbolically breaking bread in fellowship with his friends as he asked them to carry on that tradition to perpetuate selfless love, grace, kindness, compassion, and forgiveness. Profound in its simplicity.

To complement his baking meditations, Jim expanded his culinary exploits to include the art of cured meats. Jim was a deer hunter. If he was lucky enough to shoot a deer during hunting season, he would butcher the animal in our garage. Man, oh man, that garage looked like the aftermath of a bona fide massacre. Jim rigged a pully system from the rafters so he could hang the deer to execute the first phase of butchering—cleaning out the insides, pulling off the hide, beheading the animal and quartering the carcass. There was blood everywhere, with hooves, antlers and pelts from previous expeditions adorning the garage walls. Often, he'd have the grill fired up so he could cook hunks of meat fresh off the recently deceased animal while he worked. Our sons would feast like feral children, grabbing cooked meat off the grill without ceremony and gobbling it up. (Sorry vegetarians. One more reason to stick to your life choice. Am I right?) If anyone happened to amble into our garage during deer season, they'd skedaddle in a hurry because it looked like a serial killer's lair. Once the hefty first phase was done, Jim would transfer the deer parts to our basement for deboning and trimming. The whole process was complete when the cuts of meat were neatly packed in butcher paper and squirreled away in our chest freezer for use throughout the year.

Preparing venison was a skill Jim honed over time. It's a lean meat that can be easily ruined in the cooking process, but he loved both the flavor and the challenge, so he was able to summon the patience required to make delicious meals. If I close my eyes, I can taste the marsala medallions, steaks, stews and chilis that rotated through our weekly winter menu. Before he got sick, he was in the middle of making a venison soppressata. He finished that project and started curing a venison prosciutto. He continued his attention to that particular piece of meat over the course of his illness. (You may be horrified to learn that I've kept the prosciutto in my basement mini-fridge. I believe it's crossed the threshold from culinary experiment to science experiment. I just can't bring myself to throw it out.)

On the creative arts front, Jim kept pace with a number of projects. His buddy Jason answered a special request to deliver a chunk of wood from his Bristol property and carving tools so Jim could whittle a walking stick. He must've been planning ahead for when he might need a walking aid. A carved stick was more fashionable and interesting than a cane I suppose. When he wasn't carving, he was painting mini watercolors of his friends and their kids. There was a lot of industry going on in our house as we tried to stay five steps ahead of death.

Between cycles of chemo, one of Jim's friends put a bug in his ear about the virtues of parenting a potbellied pig. Apparently, this friend's daughter had one as a pet, and, as many of these stories go, she wasn't able to take it with her when she moved out so her parents became the custodians of the pig. It turns out that the guy absolutely fell in love with the pig and raved about the little guy to Jim. He was struggling with his own health issues and found the pig to be excellent company. Intrigued, Jim started researching potbellied pig adoption. All the while, Gianni cautioned that some farmers will sell you a pig, claiming that it's of the "potbellied" breed, when it's actually just a regular pig. The unsuspecting adopter doesn't figure this out until, well, the pig is bigger than what they thought it was going to be. (Sometimes I wonder if Jim had an alternate plan, à la Julia Child, if he had managed to procure a pig and it turned out to be the "wrong kind.")

Undeterred, Jim escalated his inquiry from research to pursuit. He reached out to the local humane society to see if there were any in the area. When that turned out to be a dead end, he asked our friends in rural Pennsylvania to be on the lookout for anyone selling these pigs. I eavesdropped on those conversations to gauge where he was in the process. Becoming a proud owner of a pig was *not* something I was eager to do. We already had three cats and a questionable history with other exotic animals. (Someday I'll tell you about the ball python and the baby squirrel.) But I let the whole thing play out because I wasn't going to say "No" to Jim about anything. Fortunately, (or unfortunately, depending on who you're talking to), the pig was a non-starter for the doctors. Too many germs, bacteria, etc.

You could tell the vibrancy of creation was driving both of us. We wanted things to grow, to live and to thrive. Nurturing life, even if it was just kale, felt refreshingly gratifying. In between our activities, we hung out like teenagers skipping school. We'd sit in the hot tub and chat, take naps in the living room together with our cats nestled close by or watch TV shows. We continued to walk as often as Jim felt up to it, or we took long drives out in the Finger Lakes when he didn't have the energy.

If you've never played hooky, you must drop everything and do it right now. Sneaking out of obligations and running around town having fun while everyone else is at school or work is a blast. I remember one particular day, before we had kids, when I called in sick so we could go to the opening of "Braveheart." Nothing says "hooky" like going to a weekday matinee. I can still feel the exhilaration of the little kid joy radiating through my body as we ran from the parking lot to get into the theater on time.

When my kids were school-aged, "hooky day" was part of their birthday present. They were growing up during the rapid expansion of technology so it was difficult to compete with smart phones and video games. Fortunately, the intrigue of skipping school still held enough cachet to surprise and delight them.

In the grand scheme of things, these simple experiences deliver high impact memories. The kind of memories that keep your heart company when you're lonely; that make you smile when it's raining in your soul; that warm your body in the cold and nourish the hope-maker in your brain. Go to the zoo and look at animals, go to the movies, grab a cheap lunch, or walk in the woods. Whatever it is that ignites your joy, go set it on fire for the day. You'll never get that time back again, so fuck it. Grab a loved one, or treat yourself, and go have fun. If anyone asks, tell them Jim said you could.

When we settled in at home, I could tell Jim's body was tired from waging an unrelenting war. The chemical weapon was beating the cancer back, but the toll it was taking on him was becoming much more noticeable. In addition to the chemo, there were a bunch of other drugs in his body. We began the process of weaning him off the opioids and when he was completely off the pain meds, his friends generously gifted him a grocery bag full of pot-laced baked goods to help with his nausea and ease his anxiety. I practically held vigil over the bag so our sons wouldn't decimate it for their own recreational purposes.

Mentally, Jim was weary. He wasn't used to this lack of freedom and of control over his body. "What if?" shadowed him throughout his days, adding to the drain on his psyche. A compulsion to manage certain household tasks in case he didn't get better was the undercurrent that carried him. Some were day-to-day administrative concerns, like answering the census survey and getting car insurance quotes. Larger undertakings were attended to in silent fear that he might not be able to manage them for me in the future, like paying the property tax bills for the coming year. Meanwhile, I hovered around the house like a hen aware of a fox circling the roost.

The aggressive treatments and resulting illness would eat up a good chunk of time. We enjoyed one full week home before Jim started a 10-day chemo cycle that consisted of a heavy-duty combination of Nelarabine, Cyclophosphamide, and Etoposide. For the second time, the doctor had to cut the cycle short because Jim was showing signs of encephalopathy (a broad term for brain dysfunction from any cause). His zombie-like reaction to the Nelarabine scared me more than the first go-round because I was afraid he might suffer from compounded brain damage, if that's even a thing. When I asked him a question, he might move his head to indicate that he heard me, but he wouldn't answer. I'd wait a bit, then verbally nudge him with a "Hey Hun?" I didn't want to upset him by being a pain, but I wanted to get a sense of where the edges of his waking coma were. My fear was that his brain wasn't going to fully recover from the neurotoxic effects of the chemo. Sometimes, after prompting, he'd answer in partial sentences, then disappear again. He later told me that in his head he thought he *was* answering me in real time at an appropriate, conversational speed.

It turned out my inference had been correct. Dr. B more clearly identified the link between the chemo and his mental vacation, where previously there was uncertainty on the part of the doctors as to whether or not other external factors contributed to Jim's state. She had to tweak the prescription, spreading a lower dose of Nelarabine over the course of more days rather than the high dose in a shorter span of time in order to mitigate these reactions.

The call on the play to adjust the medicines is difficult. Jim was disappointed when he had to stop the cycle because he really wanted to beat this cancer and felt this was the only chance he had. But if he kept going with the same dosing levels, he'd likely suffer permanent brain damage or die from the treatment. Dr. B knew Jim's wishes and did what she could to fight the beast while trying to reduce any negative health effects. A disturbing game of chicken between the chemo drugs and the disease ensued.

CHAPTER FOURTEEN

Covid Creep

About mid-February, I started asking the hospital nurses about Covid precautions. "Have you gotten any guidance from the hospital? Have you received any precautionary memos?" I was reading the news, and wondering why no one seemed to be alarmed. The nurses repeatedly answered in the negative. They hadn't received any memos or guidance on Corona virus protocols. As far as they knew, it wasn't a concern.

Once we were settled at home, I asked our visiting nurse if there were any extra health precautions that were being put in place to respond to the spread of the virus. She said that all the information she and her colleagues were receiving indicated that the virus wasn't going to be much worse than a bad flu, so there was no cause for alarm. The following week, she came in wearing a mask. She said the latest news from her higher-ups was that the virus was spreading, but it wasn't expected to be problematic for us. By the third week, the visiting nurse service required everyone in our household to wear masks during their visit.

That was the week a sense of urgency emerged. The remainder of March saw precautionary measures rolling out at a brisk pace. The home care protocols mirrored the hospital rules. At the Infusion Center, the evolution of the pandemic response went something like this:

> Week of 3/9/2020: Wear a mask if you're symptomatic. Wash your hands. Use hand sanitizer.
> 3/16: Doctor appointments were moved to a telemedicine format. Only necessary/emergent appointments were allowed to be in person. *Everyone* was required to wear a mask.
> 3/20: The Governor of New York shuts down nonessential movement.
> 3/23: Only one person was allowed to accompany a patient in the Cancer Center, and you had to walk directly to your appointment. You couldn't venture anywhere else.
> 3/30: The bouncers at the hospital doors were now in place behind long tables, asking a set of standardized questions and taking temperatures. "Do you feel sick? Have you been in contact with a sick person? Have you been out of the country?"

The week leading up to April 4, a guy who later tested positive for Covid lied about his symptoms so he could visit his wife and new baby in the labor wing of our hospital and the new mom got infected. Shit got serious at the hospital after that.

April fourth was the day the awful rule prohibiting anyone other than a patient from entering the hospital was instituted. That was the last day I was able to accompany Jim to his chemo treatments. What we experienced as a beehive teeming with activity one month prior now had all the eerily desolate characteristics of a morgue. A big tent was erected in the parking lot outside of the emergency room. That fucking emergency room of January 20 now looked like the scene from "E.T." where the feds show up to isolate and investigate the homesick alien. And there didn't appear to be anyone actually in the ER. The stark contrast was shocking. The previously packed parking garage I griped about earlier was now about 10% full. I could take up three parking spaces and pitch a tent if I wanted to.

The strangest part was the hospital itself. Maybe a handful of people were milling around—all keeping a healthy distance from each other. No one was coming in. Not a soul was staffing the ambassador desk. The halls were gradually being cordoned off with ropes until they were completely reduced to a narrow corral that forced single file traffic to follow tape arrows on the floor directing your movements.

We had been violently removed from our regular life in January, so this new iteration of strange manifested as nothing more than a nuisance. Though it had the potential to become seriously disruptive, I didn't have the capacity to dwell on what *might* happen if Jim needed to be readmitted to the hospital. My previous experience had taught me how important a visitor could be to augmenting care and providing much needed emotional support. The thought of him suffering alone made me physically ill, so I pushed it out of my mind. I wondered how all the sick people in the hospital were doing, like children with cancer, the frail elderly, diabetics and heart patients. The rules applied to them too. I knew the healthcare professionals were doing their best to take care of their regular patients while trying to meet the needs of the Covid-stricken. But they weren't superhuman. There would be a breaking point where prioritizations would have to be made. I didn't want to think about whose care would suffer as a result.

As logic would dictate, the correlation between Jim's diagnosis and the onset of the pandemic was coincidental. However, as I wandered through the surreal haze of our waking nightmare, it felt like they were somehow related. How could it be that the turmoil of our internal world matched that of our external world? In my momentary lapse of reason, it made sense that the entire globe stopped functioning properly to express its outrage over Jim's illness.

During the early days of the shutdown, I received reports from a friend on Long Island that she was surrounded by total mayhem. There were long lines at grocery stores and gas stations. People were losing their minds, stocking up and hunkering down. My friend urged me to get to the store and stock up because the grocery shelves by her were being cleared of everything, not just toilet paper. She was certain that it was only a matter of time before the hysteria found its way to Western New York and she was worried that, in our vulnerable state, we wouldn't be prepared.

Part of me was thinking that the hinterlands of our state never suffer as much as Metropolitan New York. While I was growing up, our crises were generally snow-related. Preparing for extended periods of time without a grocery store is part of a normal winter. Most of us keep a backstock of canned goods and pasta in our cupboards. Plus, given our current circumstance, it was really hard to elicit a deeper panic than I was already suffering.

When it came to the list of "things to be stressed about," whether or not I had a family pack of chicken thighs didn't rank high on the list. Jim was an outdoorsman. With all his supplies, we could've survived for at least a year in the wilderness. Besides, I had too much going on, and what could I possibly need that a middle-class family couldn't acquire in the United States of America? I'm embarrassed to admit that I already had about 50 rolls of Charmin. My reserve was a fluke—I hit a promotion at Target with a coupon and a gift card during a shopping trip in December. This rare trifecta of cost savings resulted in the deal of the century on toilet paper, the rare gem of spring 2020. Who could have known?

For some, the state of affairs activated a "stockpile or bust" mentality. My attitude was much different. I was looking at the world with a heightened level of empathy. While I shopped, I thought of all the people who were unable to stock up. I shopped to match our need. If Armageddon hit, there was a chest freezer full of venison in my basement and YouTube videos to teach me how to prepare it.

My hyper focus was on disinfectants. I got the jump on non-commercial cleaning agents. While people were clearing the shelves of Mr. Clean and Lysol, I stocked up on old-fashioned standards. Jugs of rubbing alcohol, peroxide, white vinegar and bleach were still available so I bought a bunch and made my own cleaning agents and sanitizers. And sanitize I did. Everything in our house. Constantly. Our doorknobs were gleaming. During the early days of the shutdown, when nothing was clear and everything was scary, my obsessive/compulsive cleaning regimen bordered on the maniacal. I swear at one point I heard my kitchen cabinets let out a squeak of fear when I returned for the 500th time, armed with my spray bottle.

In my last trip to the grocery store before my Instacarting habit began, I found the scarcity my Long Island harbinger reported. Meat cases were empty but for packages of bottom rung oddities offered up as protein alternatives. The shelves of paper products were completely empty, without even a hint of substitutes. I half expected to see an errant tumbleweed rolling down aisle seven.

Apprehension permeated the air. The few people in the store walked hurriedly past each other, casting suspicious side glances. Masks, originally worn by choice, were now mandated. Those who defiantly ignored the mask mandates clashed with the masked vigilantes. The battle of the nitwits had the potential to be entertaining if it wasn't over something so dire. When I checked out using cash, the clerk practically threw my change at me to avoid physical contact. Seemingly overnight, we were living a Netflix new release.

After that dreadful shopping trip, my grocery store visits were decidedly over. I finally gave in and embraced the wonders of Instacart. Initially, I approached the process with reluctance and a modicum of distrust. Grocery shopping had been a major weekly event throughout my adult life. Handing the actual shopping trip responsibility over to another person felt strange. What if they messed up my order? Is it going to be too expensive? It turned out that the convenience vastly outweighed my misgivings. After one delivery, I was a total convert. I didn't care one iota if I got something I didn't intend. And the cost? Worth every stinkin' penny. I think I actually saved money—or at least it was a wash—because I wasn't impulse buying.

Simultaneously, Grubhub factored prominently in our household food forage. Jim's food tolerance was ever changing. It was easier to order from multiple restaurants through Grubhub than to try and make something that would satisfy a cancer patient and two young men. Our friends had been cheering us on from the sidelines of our cancer battle and asking for assignments to help ease our burden. I finally put the word out on CaringBridge that Grubhub gift certificates were the most useful support we could have. I'll never forget the moment after I pressed "post" on my request. A torrent of Grubhub gift certificates came flooding into my email inbox. I felt like I was watching a Vegas lottery machine. I burst into tears at the overwhelming response. I didn't realize how many people were waiting and wanting to help. Thanks to our exceptionally generous friends and family, we were in rich supply of Grubhub certificates throughout Jim's illness. It's amazing how much love and warmth you can feel from afar.

Jim's immunosuppression brought a myriad of restrictions to socializing. When Covid emerged, the meager number of visits we could engage in was completely eliminated. The inability to host friends and family was a mixed blessing. Without the clear boundaries set by the pandemic, I imagined our home would have been a revolving door of guests, despite the physicians' cautions. Jim was an exceptional extrovert, which at times could be a point of contention in our marriage. His constant need to fill all his time with people and activity clashed with my preference for the peace and quiet of our home and the pleasure of his company. Now, I finally had him all to myself, but what a shitty reason. It sucked, not only because he would have enjoyed the distraction but because he would have liked to have seen more people before he passed away.

The precautions made visits to Jim's mom very stressful. They wanted to see each other regularly, but we were afraid that one would unknowingly infect the other. Jim was in and out of the hospital and his mother was still visiting with friends and family. The few times we made it over to her house, we wore our masks and sat across the dining room from her. The combination of masks, distance and an elderly woman's impaired hearing made conversations unsatisfying.

I hated being the enforcer, especially when it came to Jim's mom. I felt like a human barrier preventing the healing salve of human contact from being shared between mother and son. Contact might cause deadly infections, but the lack of contact meant the absence of one of the best means to alleviate heartache. Keeping them physically apart was counterintuitive to all of us. But the whole pandemic seemed like such a gamble, and we'd already lost big on the cancer lottery. When a lump formed in my throat watching the two of them longing to close the distance, terror outweighed my desire to ditch the rules.

The social drought compounded Jim's psychological strain. The "What-the-Fuck-edness" of it all was staggering. The virus was proving to be wily, spreading around the globe like wildfire. People were dying at an alarming rate, yet no one knew much about it. Daily reports from various government officials were unclear, contradictory, and downright confusing. The default defense against illness was isolation.

As a family, we had to make important decisions about the living arrangements for our sons. One of our decisions was made for us. Though most people's lives were turned upside down by college closings, ours was eased by this welcome turn of events. Gianni wasn't very happy at college, and I imagine the added worry about his father weighed heavily on him. He was already making the worrisome two-hour drive along Lake Erie twice a week in wintry conditions so he could spend time with Jim. We were thrilled to welcome him home for his virtual learning experience.

Giacomo was going to school locally, working at two restaurants, and sharing an apartment with two other people who frequented New York City. With his level of public exposure, the kid was a walking petri dish. He became quite sick during the month of February with some kind of respiratory something-or-other that wouldn't go away. Once he was through the worst part of it, he continued to visit his father. In hindsight, it might have been Covid, but we'll never know. I'm embarrassed to say that his illness didn't register with me because I was so focused on Jim. My maternal instincts were on vacation. The most I could do was harp on him to observe all the CDC precautions while I followed him around with a can of Lysol.

The community pool

Maybe it was the new clarity with which I was seeing the world now that Jim was fighting for his life, but it seemed like during the spring of 2020, life and death were tied together more closely than I'd ever experienced. Our spring continued to unfold in May with all the poetic trappings of a Disney movie. The weather was sunny and beautiful. The bulbs and early spring flowers were coming up unencumbered by late-season snows. The colors were brilliant, and the cacophony of animal mating rituals was borderline obscene. Our city felt like a Hollywood production. This was the kind of spring that us Western New Yorkers long for but rarely get due to late March snow squalls, and snow and cold spells continuing into April.

This exquisite season was the backdrop to our struggles with cancer and the Covid pandemic. Pictures of an empty Times Square and an LA without cars looked fake. Workers sent home to Zoom were freaking out. I was starting to hear about friends who were sick with Covid as fear spread across the country like smog.

At this bizarre intersection of life and death, a spirited social scene evolved across the street from our house in the school parking lot. Sent home from college and unable to work, an outsized number of young adults found themselves with an abundance of free time on their hands. Our sons attended their virtual classes, but let's face it, in the early days of tele-learning academic rigor was nonexistent. They hovered around home to do their schoolwork and to hang out with Jim, but it wasn't mentally healthy for them to be immersed in cancer all the time. Unfortunately, everyone's choices were severely limited. They boiled down to: 1. Stay home, or 2. Go outside and play while wearing a mask and maintaining a six-foot buffer zone between you and everyone else.

In normal times, the neighborhood kids used the school lot for skateboarding after the teachers were gone for the day. Now that schools were shut down, the parking lot was wide open and without restriction. Giacomo was a die-hard skater boy. As the walls of the pandemic began to close in, he was out there practicing his "Ollies" and "Kick Turns" on the regular. Gianni wasn't a big skater, but he was bored so he went out there with his brother. By the end of March, their buddy Aedan was back in town and joined them. The three guys spent countless hours, showing off their mad skills and goofing off. Any time Jim and I needed a little levity, we would peek out the living room window to watch their antics.

As the pandemic plodded on, an increasing number of people joined in on the fun. Simultaneously, in the schoolyard adjacent to the parking lot, a handful of neighbors started meeting regularly with their dogs, creating an unofficial dog park. Before we knew it, the schoolyard had evolved into a socially distanced neighborhood gathering spot. I started referring to the lot as the "community pool" because it reminded me of my childhood days when kids hung out all day at our local recreation center. The convenience of proximity became apparent as Jim's illness progressed. The boys were a short call-across-the-yard away if we needed help with anything. Even more remarkable was the fact that, of all the parking lots in Rochester, these young adults whose lives were suspended in the most extraordinary way chose to gather in front of our house. Without prescription or agenda, they showed up for our sons, and by association, for us. With all the hardship they were enduring, to squeak joy out of the hand they were dealt, these kids embodied optimism. They reminded me of water lilies growing out of the mud.

Fever

In the first two weeks of April, Jim went through another 10-day cycle of chemotherapy. His strength was a marvel. The compounded exposure to these strong chemicals was knocking the hell out of him, but he still rallied to make homemade manicotti on Easter Sunday. My family gathered together for Easter via zoom. We played show and tell with our respective meals, then parted ways to watch Andre Bocelli's broadcast concert, *Music for Hope*, live from the Duomo in Milan. The virtual connection with family felt more meaningful than some of our previous in-person get-togethers. The intentional effort we put into gathering remotely conveyed the loving embrace we all desperately needed. The high-energy buzz that typically accompanied our family gatherings was muted by zoom, making way for the beauty of a stripped-down version of ourselves.

Though Jim fought with the might of giants, he couldn't elude the deleterious effects of the chemo. The day after Easter, he fainted after coming up the stairs too quickly. He had fallen asleep on the couch, and I had decided not to rouse him when I retired to bed. This was one of those moments when my vigilance was impaired by exhaustion. Gianni was downstairs with Jim in case he needed anything. Jim woke up with a start. Feeling a little disoriented, his mind focused on going upstairs to bed while his body wasn't ready for the brisk activity. He got to our bedroom door and promptly fainted. Thank God he didn't hit his head or break a leg. I bundled him off to bed and talked to the nurses the next day about changing out one of his medications. To see him so vulnerable created an indescribable ache in my heart.

In the middle of all of this, when I didn't think my nerves could be tested further, Jim came down with a fever. God, I'm still mad at myself for being overly cautious. He felt warm to me so I took his temperature and it was 100.8. Jim didn't want me to call the Center because he absolutely did not want to go back into the hospital. But everything I read and everything we were told said "If Jim has a fever, call the Center!" Ugh, I should've realized that it was just his hat. One of our neighbors knitted him this hat that he loved to wear. If I had taken his hat off and waited a half hour, I'm sure the temperature would have been gone. But instead, I sided with the kind of caution driven by overzealous fear. I called the doctor and, as you'd expect, they said "Bring him in."

Hospital entry protocols were totally different since we first started this odyssey. Pre-Covid, Jim would have gone straight to the Cancer Center for assessment. If everything was okay, he would have been released in a day. With the new rules in place, Jim had to go through the emergency room, adding an additional day to his stay. I drove up to the E.T. tent and was greeted by two unfriendly men guarding the entrance. I had to let Jim out in the parking lot and watch him walk into that stark homage to some dystopian novel. Because he was a cancer patient, they put him in a room by himself, where he waited for hours until someone could administer a Covid test. Then he had to wait even longer for the results. They finally admitted him to the Cancer Center that night. Of course, as soon as he walked into the ER, the fever was gone and never came back. He was pretty pissed off about the whole scene. I got an earful when he got released 48 hours later. But, truthfully? It was probably the best thing for both of us at the time. The doctors kept an eye on him for a couple days and I got a little break. From that day forward, if we disagreed on something, he'd ask me if I was going to call the Cancer Center and tell them he was running a fever. Apparently, chemo didn't eliminate his wise-assery.

Throughout his false-alarm stay, I wasn't allowed in the hospital. Our desire to be together, for better or for worse, faced an enemy. The implications vis-à-vis Jim's potential need for critical care and possible end-of-life support twisted my stomach. Covid was fast becoming more than a nuisance.

A young sales clerk summed up these forced separations best in three words. She told me her mother-in-law passed away in a nursing home and that her husband wasn't allowed in, so he had to say "Goodbye" via facetime. Distressed by the retelling of the story, she struggled to find the right words to describe the inexplicable. I'll never forget her profound reflection: "It was gross." My heart sank. In one month, our wealthy, intelligent country had been brought to its knees, leaving us all witless and unable to humanely aid our most vulnerable. Gross.

No retreat, no surrender

When Jim returned from his brief hospital stay, he reported that his hair was falling out in earnest. Apparently, it was coming out in clumps so he wanted to shave it all off post haste. He didn't look mangy to me. I thought he could wait a little longer, but he was adamant. Perhaps he wanted to shave it himself as a way of wrestling control out of chemo's hands. His great head of hair symbolized youthful vibrancy. If it had to go, he was going to do it on his own terms, staking a claim in the battle for his body on any ground he could gain. Even if it was a hollow victory, it was worth the temporary feeling of control.

I objected to the shearing and gently tried to persuade him to wait. I dreaded the Telly Savalas look because baldness would be an inescapable reminder that there was an unwelcome guest wreaking havoc in his body. People with cancer can look very healthy right up until their hair falls out. A naked head announces "CANCER!" like a carnival barker betraying your condition before you can open your mouth to say "Hi." Throughout the first couple months of Jim's illness, I tried to keep him from looking like a cancer patient by bringing him café casual clothes and helping him attend to his personal grooming. I was pushing back on the invasion, saying "No!" to the marauder at the gate. If Jim didn't look like he was sick, then maybe we could trick the illness into thinking it was in the wrong body.

We were in the kitchen with all the necessary tools, discussing Jim's hair while our sons milled about, energizing us with the brightness of their youth. Realizing Jim was firm on his intentions, I quietly laid my objections to rest and mentally prepared myself to support Jim's wishes. Though I wasn't ready to succumb to this symbolic ritual, I executed it with levity and encouragement. My husband, ever a paragon of strength, was attacking the unknown with dignity and bravery. Marveling at his tenacity, I rallied and joined him on the battle field with clippers in hand—chin up and chest puffed. I realized that through this act, we weren't giving in. Shaving Jim's head in the kitchen—the heart of our home—was a call to arms. It was time for us to dig a little deeper and unite our strength as a family to fortify the ramparts against our encroaching foe.

As I started shaving Jim's head, a cold wind howled in my soul while love swelled up in my chest. The complicated feelings I was experiencing awakened my whole self to the reality of life's paradox that the agony and ecstasy of love are intertwined. The universe offers this enigmatic gift again and again in a variety of forms. Whether it's in the eyes of your infant gazing up at you, your friend's hug, or the love of your life's shaved head, there is an open invitation to love all around us. But if we choose to open our hearts, pain walks in hand in hand as love's "plus one."

When the barbering was over, I gave Jim a hand mirror while the boys came closer to inspect my handiwork. In that moment, I felt the love of our family grow deeper because of our pain. All four of us were in this together. No one hid. No one was giving up. Together, we were strong. Together, we were facing the storm. Together we all knew that life must come to an end and the only thing that mattered was the love we shared. Feeling the weight of our reality, we boldly stood in solidarity with brave hearts, silently committing to our future. No retreat. No surrender.

CHAPTER FIFTEEN

See-Saw Margery Daw

While we struggled to achieve remission, any conversation we had with Jim's oncology team fell into the "difficult" category. They did their best to help us interpret cancer's road signs while balancing our need to feel some hope. Dr. B and her nurses were honest with us as we all paddled through the troubled waters. It's professionally responsible to be forthcoming with the truth, but that doesn't make it any less painful for them. I could see it in their eyes. And we weren't the only people on their dance card in the terminal illness ballroom. We were fortunate to be in the care of these gifted human beings who were as kind as they were smart. They guided us through Jim's cancer treatments like naval captains through a minefield.

The month started with an aggressive, 10-day treatment cycle. Dr. B was walking that fine line of trying to beat the cancer out of Jim while simultaneously minimizing long-term damage to his body. The ass-kicking regimen left him feeling like hell for the better part of the month. Earnest transplant conversations commenced in the middle of Jim's chemo beating. Dr. B recommended the procedure as an important next step in his long haul to cure, *if* we could get his cancer in remission. No one knew whether or not remission would be achieved, so it was difficult to put our minds into that space. However, if we *were* successful in achieving remission, Dr. B believed that having a bone marrow transplant (a.k.a. BMT) was our only chance at preventing the return of the cancer. In the event Jim was able to take that route, time was of the essence. They wanted to execute a transplant before the cancer came back, and a number of steps had to be completed to prepare Jim for the procedure.

To further explore the option, we met with the BMT doctor assigned to Jim. His notes from our meeting speak for themselves:

> *"We discussed that if he achieves a complete remission with chemotherapy, he likely has a 30–50% three-year overall survival with transplant, but if he continues to have a partial remission, odds of a favorable outcome fall to the five-to-thirty percent range and we would have to discuss the pros and cons of proceeding with transplant in this scenario. If he has continued partial response, we can discuss the utility of a second cycle of NCE prior to transplant versus referring him to another center like Baylor for a clinical trial of anti CD5 or CD7 CAR-T therapy."*

It wasn't a very hopeful conversation. Taking the transplant route was predicated on remission, but fate was keeping a stiff poker face. Without much else to go on, we remained cautiously optimistic and proceeded with transplant preparations.

Growing up, I was a high-energy little kid. As you'd expect with any high energy little kid, I absolutely HATED school.

And school hated me. My grammar schooling took place in the '70s—an era when no one knew or cared about ADHD, dyslexia, or any of the other "different" ways a kid could process information. Trouble was my constant companion because I could not focus or sit still. This terrible combination spiraled into a vicious cycle of acting out, getting in trouble, stewing with feelings of guilt and shame, getting distracted then starting again. Recess was the only relief I felt in a day that was one big pressure cooker. You could practically hear the steam engine whistle blowing out my ears when I finally got to go outside and run around.

Do you remember playground seesaws? Teeter-tottering was one of my favorite activities. A whole-body experience that was perfect for my vibrating mind and body. The sensory stimulation started with the feeling of the ground beneath my feet while my fingers curled around the cold metal handles. I'd position myself with anticipation like a frog ready to leap from her lily pad. Then, the strong and purposeful spring through my legs, lifting off from the earth, aiming for the ozone! I wanted to get lift and speed enough to capture that woozy feeling of elevation in my chest. In that brief apex moment, there was a magnificent floaty feeling that quickly transformed into tummy butterflies on the way down. My feet switched rolls from catapult to cushion, softly welcoming me back down to earth. Aaaahhh. Finally, some peace to replace my feeling of failure, if only for a little while.

The seesaw offered both personal respite and cool physics lessons about balance and gravity as more kids piled on to each side. The game shifted seamlessly from a two-person event to a team sport. Exhilarating! Many of you listening are cringing right about now because you're familiar with the cruel social lesson seesaws taught us about trust. Who can forget the fated day your seesaw partner made the sinister decision to jump off their end, sending you crashing down to break your keister. I can still feel that awful jolt through my spine.

When I think about our deliberations over whether or not to pursue the transplant, it kind of felt like all the doctors were on one side of the seesaw, holding their end down, while our family dangled up in the air, unsure if we were going to crash or float down.

Based on the aggressive nature of Jim's leukemia, it was a forgone conclusion that if forced into remission, the disease would rally to spring back like a Hydra. The two treatment options available to respond to this seeming inevitability were maintenance chemotherapy or BMT. Judging from the fact that the cancer was undeterred by previous treatments, we figured the maintenance chemo regimen would be rigorous and likely foiled by the leukemia. By what amount of time Jim's life would be prolonged with maintenance, no one would say, but our team emphasized BMT in our options discussions, so we figured maintenance wasn't going to be an effective long-term solution. If and when the cancer returned, a "Hail Mary" BMT would no longer be an option, which meant Jim would transition to comfort care as we braced ourselves for his final days.

The BMT option was much more invasive and rigorous than maintenance chemotherapy, but gave Jim fifty-fifty odds of beating the disease. Coin-toss odds, when it comes to your life, suck. Even if we came up with a successful transplant, Jim's future did not look great. The cancer would likely shadow him until it returned within three to five years like an uninvited drunk uncle at Thanksgiving. Remission would bring a continuous parade of doctors' appointments, blood draws and bone scans. Jim's activities and interests would be scaled way back. Spectating at the things he loved to do as a full participant would drive him insane. As a couple, our roles as patient and caregiver would be solidified, affecting the power dynamic in our relationship. And we can't forget the Covid factor. Living as a permanently immunocompromised person, Jim's social butterfly wings would be clipped. (I could hear our arguments over Covid care echoing through my imagined scenarios.) None of that sounded optimal, but the *possibility* remained that Jim could have a little more time with us if the procedure was successful. *If* was the siren song floating in the air, beckoning us as we weighed the options.

I read somewhere that the average adult makes about 35,000 decisions a day, and that 90% of those are made by our subconscious. It's the larger decisions that grab the attention of our consciousness. Generally speaking, one's deliberation process relies on information based on one's own experience, acquired knowledge and input from content experts. Working out all this information to arrive at an optimal solution takes place against the backdrop of one's setting—a highly influential element that is often out of our control.

With regard to personal experience, all Jim and I had was a list of friends and family who had died of cancer. Not being science-y types, three decades of watching PBS and blind research on the internet filled in our acquired knowledge, while the majority of our information came from the doctors. As we understood it, to BMT or not to BMT boiled down to: If you don't do it, you're gonna die soon. If you go through with it, you might die a little later. We weren't in an optimal state of mind to think through the imagined scenarios. Over the arc of

Jim's illness, he endured extreme illness, crisis, fear, sadness, excruciating pain, social isolation, stress, exhaustion, and anger, while plagued with worries about his family, home, and money. Throw on that tire fire our complex grief of mourning a vibrant life curtailed while anticipatory grief invited ruminations over the possibility of a life soon to end. It makes sense that one's executive function might experience partial paralysis as a result of this extreme overload. Just try and feel confident about any decision you make under these conditions, let alone one where life and death hang in the balance.

And what about the setting? Well, my friends, that is what has kept a decent campfire burning in the backyard of my mind for over two years. Under non-pandemic conditions, a typical hospital vibrates with freneticism. They are not calm relaxing environments in which to make serious decisions. The pandemic escalated that vibe to levels unseen by even the most seasoned emergency management and critical care veterans.

As our minds struggled under this weight, we reviewed what was being presented to us. In the transplant column, activity was poppin'. The nurse coordinator laid out an overwhelming schedule of doctor appointments, tests, and procedures. For some reason, running around with lots of activity makes us feel useful in the face of a situation that is way out of our control. To enhance the gratification that diligent industry delivers, all the action items had to be completed in a tight timeframe, leaving little room to stop, breathe, and think between procedures. The maintenance column was sparsely populated with action items, few people were involved, and there weren't any manmade timelines to speak of. Just life taking its natural course. You might think the potential curative properties of the BMT side heavily outweighed the maintenance side as the focus of our decision-making calculus. And you would be right. We adopted an "If we're busy, we must be making progress." mindset.

Having had time to think about it, I now realize that the maintenance side, with but a few to-do items, was markedly more significant than the BMT side from a psychological perspective. Maintenance would warrant our full attention, crowding out thoughts of deep conversations about quality of life, core values, spiritual needs, and end-of-life preparations. But we all avoided those conversations like one would avoid a bloated deer carcass on a 90-degree day. The maintenance option didn't fit the culture model of our treating facility, or that of society as a whole.

We had plenty of content experts to advise, inform, and consult for the transplant who were all at the ready to spring into the stratosphere from their position on the seesaw. But there weren't any professionals on the maintenance side trained in holding space to support the deeper conversations that would have better prepared us for what was to come. In fact, there was one crucial team that was glaringly absent from our entire cancer journey. A team that many learned minds argue is as important as the oncology team. I'm referring to the psychosocial health care professionals. These are the folks who view the patient as a whole person, and who would have put Jim squarely in the center of the patient experience from the very beginning.

CHAPTER SIXTEEN

Psychosocial Support

What is psychosocial support? When someone is diagnosed with cancer, their life is tossed on its head. Even an emotionally solid, psychologically balanced, spiritually grounded person is going to experience some level of trauma when learning that life as they knew it is forever changed for the worse. Depending on the type and severity of the cancer, a patient may also be faced with the existential crisis ignited by a terminal diagnosis. Despite Jim's positive disposition, he was not immune to the effects of situational depression.

Psychosocial teams collaborate with patients and families to meet their mental, emotional, social, and spiritual needs. For cancer patients, these teams are often led by a psychosocial oncologist, and are made up of any combination of clinical social workers trained specifically to provide a therapeutic experience, psychologists, and faith-based professionals. Some cancer centers weave these teams in equally with the oncology teams. They are proactive in nature and recognize that a life-altering diagnosis can cause significant distress for patients and their families, which in turn, can have a negative impact on the patient's health outcomes.

When you think of it, grief counselors are among the first responders called upon by local municipalities and school systems to support those traumatized by large-scale acts of violence. The counselors' role is to help folks process their trauma and grief. Without proactive mental health support, many people affected by crises internalize their trauma. That coping strategy, though seemingly effective at first, chips away at one's physical and emotional health.

The violent act Jim suffered wasn't perpetrated by an external foe. Jim's own body turned on him. From the moment we walked into the emergency room, we were pummeled with a series of life-altering realities and traumatic events. Having a trained therapeutic professional in our corner throughout our cancer odyssey would have helped us better cope and care for ourselves and each other. As a patient, it's important to have your thoughts and feelings validated. Being seen and heard is empowering, and can transform your self-perception from one of patient-victim to patient-partner. The top-down power balance between patient and doctors shifts to a truly patient-centered experience where the patient is an equal participant, collaborating with the medical teams in their own care. If you have that support throughout your cancer experience, the fingers of panic that are gripping your brain tend to loosen, so you start to feel like you have agency over what's happening to you.

If Jim had had the support of trained psychosocial clinicians from the moment Dr. B delivered her diagnosis, when the bone marrow transplant tidal wave came our way, we might have paused that wave in midair to create the space for a more thorough conversation about the maintenance option. We also might have paid closer attention to the fact that, on the day before Jim was scheduled to enter the hospital to start the bone marrow transplant process, he felt an ache in his lower back. It had been four weeks since his last chemo treatment. Was the cancer back again, rendering the upcoming transplant useless? When Jim told his doctors that he was experiencing this pain, no one stopped to contemplate what his body was telling everyone. Was this our version of the Challenger's "O" rings?

I can't help but think that there was an unspoken culture in our cancer center that cultivated an attitude of: "If he's cured, then everything will be okay. And if not? He'll be dead and it won't matter." A cold, clinical culture would explain why they left psychosocial care up to the patients and their families. To me, that's the same as leaving the *cancer treatments* up to the families. We don't know what we don't know. How are we supposed to evaluate what we're grappling with? How are we to know what questions to ask or what's normal and what type of mental health care to seek out?

It is a choice made by a healthcare facility's leadership not to incorporate psychosocial care into the treatment plans of its patients. I think there are a couple of factors that go into this wrongheaded approach. First and foremost, the choice is financially-driven, not patient-driven. Time is money. The hospital and insurance companies put a price tag on every minute a healthcare professional spends with a patient. Insurance companies barely cover mental health support, which means the hospital would have to budget to cover the cost of care and likely bill the patient. This clearly wasn't a direction our cancer center leadership was interested in going.

And speaking of money, we can't deny the fact that Jim's treatments generated a decent amount of revenue for the cancer center. That's quite jaded, isn't it? But not unfounded. A 2022 Wall Street Journal article titled *Profit from America's Healthcare Bloat* reported:

> "In the US, everyone from your primary-care doctor to your cardiologist has an incentive to make you consume as much healthcare as possible, from the prescription drug you could do without to the expensive surgical procedure you might be able to avoid through physical therapy." (David Wainer, "Profit from America's Healthcare Bloat." Wall Street Journal, 9/4/22).

While Jim's treatments could generate a profit for the hospital, non-reimbursable care like psychosocial support would eat into their margin. To make matters worse, at the time Jim's BMT was being discussed by his medical team, our treating hospital was reportedly losing over $130 million a month in clinical revenue alone, (compliments of the coronavirus.) That meant Jim, with his decent health insurance and multiple approvals for potentially life-saving care, was one big fat cash cow.

Another consideration is our culture's inability to discuss death and dying in a healthy way, so we avoid it like dog poop on the sidewalk. Though doctors face death every day, it doesn't make them any more comfortable talking about it. If you have a dog, and walk it daily, you don't gleefully pick up the product of its colon. No lie here. In this day and age, many doctors still won't tell their terminal patients that they are dying. Looking someone in the eyes and telling them the truth about their prognosis while they're surrounded by their loved ones is painful. Doctors are humans too.

To exacerbate the situation, many doctors internalize the loss of a patient as a personal failure. Whether it's on a conscious level or not, the idea that they've failed lives somewhere in their brains. That's an uncomfortable feeling to be avoided—much like dog poop.

Finally, the stigma assigned to mental illness feeds a general lack of understanding regarding what mental health care actually consists of, and when and why it's needed. Conversations about mental health typically make people as uncomfortable as talking about death, but in a different way. General misunderstanding and a profound lack of education on mental health and psychosocial support leaves many feeling like outcasts and acts as a huge barrier to treatment. We aren't good emotional communicators in our culture. We still suffer the vestiges of a post WWII era attitude that doesn't recognize mental health as "a thing." "Suck it up, get over it and keep it to yourself" is our prevailing attitude toward mental health.

Our family was unknowingly caught up in the vortices of these factors when I initiated requests for support. In the early days of cancer, Jim and I both recognized that what he was experiencing was too much for one person to handle. At the time, we didn't know there was such a thing as psychosocial support, so I inquired about mental health counseling. Though related, there is a difference between the two. Mental health supports are reactive, and provided to patients who have a mental health diagnosis identified by the *Diagnostic and Statistical Manual of Mental Disorders* like manic depression, suicidal ideation, or schizophrenia. Services are provided by the psychiatric department in response to a request from the treating physician. The focus is on the patient and doesn't account for the family unit or context of a situation.

Psychosocial support is a proactive approach to supporting an otherwise mentally healthy person as they face a major disruption in their lives. In this case, a cancer diagnosis. The strategies seek to support the patient and their family with a psychotherapeutic experience throughout the course of their illness journey. An emphasis on *seeing* patients rather than *watching* them gives the patient a sense of control in an expressly out of control environment. Because this type of care is preventive and more nuanced than reactive mental health care, many don't understand what it is. Given the distinction, it makes sense that my inquiries were met with avoidance and vague responses from nurses with averted eyes. They didn't have anything to offer by way of mental health counseling in the cancer center, so they pointed me to the social worker on the floor.

The social worker gave me a list of flimsy programs that were off-site. Why yes, you are correct in observing that Jim was in critical condition and not going to be released from the hospital any time soon. That was it. There was no other offering or effort to understand what we needed. I had my hands, head, and heart full, so I wasn't going on a crusade to demand attention. Besides, it seemed like I was speaking a language that no one at the cancer center understood.

Our treating facility had their pants around their ankles when it came to patient-centered care. We experienced sympathy and, at times, empathy. But those polite human responses rank high on the list of platitudes, sharing equal space with "thoughts and prayers." Yes, Jim's body was attended to, but, emotionally, he was left to his own devices to walk through the heart of darkness.

I don't know, man. It was hard to wrap my head around it when I learned that our hospital, the University of Rochester Medical Center, is home to the original biopsychosocial model. The Model is a multi-disciplinary theory of illness and healing, developed in 1977 by internist and psychiatrist George Libman Engel. Without getting too far into the weeds, the biopsychosocial model postulates that to understand a person's medical condition, attending physicians need to take into account the biological factors, *and* the psychological and social factors. The approach emphasizes the critical role of the patient's environment and mental health in diagnosing illness and determining treatment.

The biopsychosocial approach to patient care was highlighted more recently by the former CEO of our treating hospital, Dr. Bradford Berck. In 2021, Dr. Berck published his book: *Getting your Brain & Body Back: Everything You Need to Know after Spinal Cord Injury, Stroke, or Traumatic Brain Injury*. Dr. Berck suffered an acute neurological injury (ANI) from a tragic bicycling accident in 2009. His brilliant book is a "how-to" narrative for people recovering from an ANI. In a nod to the biopsychosocial model, Dr. Berk devotes the first chapter to the importance of managing your mental health in the face of a tragic, life-altering ANI diagnosis. I submit that Dr. Berk's incorporation of mental health care in a total patient care model can and should be applied to any patient receiving a life-altering diagnosis.

This holistic approach to patient care benefits the physicians and nurses as well. Therapists dedicated to supporting the social emotional health of their patients relieve pressure on the doctors who must continuously deliver difficult news. If the doctors know there is a trained professional supporting their patients' emotional health, they are freed up to focus on the physical part of patient care without being afraid of receiving a patient reaction that they aren't trained or prepared to handle. (Think of the doctor who unceremoniously told us back in February that there was nothing more they could do for Jim.)

Coming up empty from our treating physicians, I supported Jim the only way I knew how—I threw open every single portal I could think of to let the love of friends and family pour in. The support lifted his spirits to a degree, as did finally getting to go home. But as we waded into the next phase of treatments, the soothing balm of love gradually lost its effectiveness against the onslaught of the disease and treatments while the shadows of depression loomed large.

CHAPTER SEVENTEEN

Zero Minus Five

In the five or so weeks since Jim had been released from the hospital, we had grown accustomed to the tender care of our outpatient oncology team and relished our time at home. But we could feel the undercurrents generated by the transplant team picking up speed, carrying us further and further away from our comfort zone.

Jim was assigned a nurse coordinator to get him properly prepared to move forward if his cancer went into remission. Working in tandem with our oncology team, Nurse G oversaw all Jim's tests, procedures, and appointments. The transplant preparation checklist was long and daunting, considering the tight timeframe. A sense of urgency was pulsing beneath the surface of her clinical demeanor.

The most important step in the preparation process was finding a bone marrow donor match, which is difficult and takes time. The team starts searching for one as soon as they think the procedure is a possibility. They comb the national bone marrow donor registry while simultaneously testing selected family members. In our case, they came up empty-handed from the registry.

After testing our sons and the younger of Jim's two brothers (age is a factor in transplant success rates, thus automatically eliminating Jim's oldest brother), they found both our sons to be 50% matches. We were told that studies found that 50% matches worked just as well as 100% matches. This was good news because we didn't need to wait for a match like so many others before us. We had one built in.

Based on the science of success, 20-year-old Gianni was selected for his younger blood. The process dictated that Gianni go to the cancer center for five consecutive days to receive shots that would help excite stem cell growth and speed up their entry into his blood stream. On the sixth day, Gianni's blood would be removed through an IV line. The part of the white blood cells that contains stem cells would be separated in a machine and given to Jim. The red blood cells would then be returned to Gianni.

This physical sacrifice was a beautiful gift to give his father. But we were worried this act of selflessness carried an emotional burden. Though the procedure isn't painful, it is daunting. Both our kids were fully caught up in the strange world of distance learning and Covid restrictions while watching their father suffer. As "the match" for 50/50 odds, I couldn't help but think of the additional emotional stress Gianni would be carrying about potential failure. And what about Giacomo—the one who didn't get chosen? Were there feelings there? Cancer was now messing with my whole family in an eerily vampiric way.

On April 24, Jim's oncologist called to say that the recent scans showed the mass in his chest was shrinking. Finally, some good news. Several days later, she called back with even *better* news. The results we'd all been waiting for. *Zero* leukemic cells were found in the biopsy sample. Wow! We could hardly believe it. After everything Jim had gone through, this was wonderful to hear. Reveling in the "all clear" didn't last long. Now that they had the green light, the transplant team went full tilt getting Jim and Gianni ready for the procedure.

Prior to the procedure, several friends offered to connect Jim with transplant survivors. The well-intentioned wanted Jim to hear positive stories about trial, tribulation, and triumph. But he declined those invitations. In order to force himself through the doorway leading to yet another level of hell, he needed to wrap himself up in as much emotional insulation as possible. Speaking to predecessors contained a possibility of upsetting his denial, which was a tremendous tool for his brain to use to help him cope with the overwhelming nature of his situation.

Buddhists remind us that suffering is an inescapable part of life. The universe teases us with the fact that we don't get to choose our suffering, only our response. As demons dangled Jim off a precipice overlooking perdition, he had to squint his eyes and blur the imminent agony to focus on the tiny twinkle of hope calling from the other side of the chasm. The boys and I joined him in avoidance by huddling behind our own parapets. None of us knew just how bad the aftereffects of killing all of Jim's nascent cells was going to be. We were hopeful for cure and recovery. We couldn't consider anything else.

On Mother's Day, I dropped my husband and my son off at cancer camp. I watched them approach the sliding glass doors—two men embarking on a hero's journey. Jim carried his mandolin while Gianni wheeled a large suitcase containing everything Jim would need for one month's stay. *Everything but me,* I thought. As they disappeared into the building, I envisioned a deep moat around the cancer center carved out by Covid.

Over the years, I've waved from our porch with love and pride as I watched my family set out on their adventures together. Whether they were trudging along on their daily trek to school or pulling out of the driveway with a strategically packed Pontiac Vibe on a camping adventure, the electricity of excitement and anticipation lit them up. As mother and wife, it lit *me* up to see my guys spending important father-son time together.

This time, nausea held court in my stomach as I watched Jim and Gianni disappear into the cancer center. Concerned for their health, safety, and emotional wellbeing, I was afraid of what was to come. Yet there was something comforting about watching them walk in together. They were embarking on a different kind of journey. One filled with apprehension rather than joy. But they had each other, and that gave them the courage to proceed.

Cancer treatments are given in cycles, and the days in the cycle are numbered. What those cycles and numbers are depends on your prescription. In the case of Jim's bone marrow transplant, day zero was the day Jim received Gianni's blood. The prep days leading up to day zero are counted out in the negative. Mother's Day for example was minus five. On that day, Gianni received his first in the series of shots while Jim was admitted and got hit with his first chemo treatment of the cycle. In the next three days, (days minus 4, minus 3, and minus 2), I would bring Gianni to the cancer center for his shots while Jim was blasted with more chemo and two daily courses of total body irradiation. On day minus one, Gianni went in for six hours of blood collection. Later that day, Jim would be infused with Gianni's healthy, hopeful blood. From there, the medical team would keep a close eye on Jim—looking to see if Gianni's blood would regenerate properly in place of the fucked up leukemic cells.

The medical team estimated Jim would be able to come home after 30 days. That sounded like such a long time to be apart while your person is suffering. We'd been together for 30 years. In that time, we'd never been apart for more than a week. It was like some kind of penance we had to pay—one day per year. There was nothing else to do but trust the process and the professionals.

Making love

During the months leading up to Jim's second hospitalization, our love-making was throttled back—for obvious reasons. Navigating around all we were dealing with would dampen anyone's sex drive. Jim's body was fighting a 360-degree war. Though he started his battle from a position of strength, four months of treatments had taken their toll. I myself didn't initiate sex because I was tired, worried all the time, and afraid of hurting him. Jim felt fragile to me.

An additional, unexpected barrier to physical intimacy manifested in a side effect of one of the chemo drugs. It's widely known that chemotherapy can cause a condition called neuropathy, which is a type of nerve damage. Symptoms include weakness, numbness, and pain in the extremities. What is not widely known is that the chemo drug Vincristine raises the neuropathy ante by interfering with the nerves and vasculature that control erections.

After the initial rounds of chemo in January, Jim had been bothered by a strange sensation in his penis. He had difficulty describing the feeling, and I had difficulty understanding because, well, I don't have a penis. Dr. B came in to talk with him about it. He proceeded to describe the feeling as a constant pressure—like his penis was becoming erect out of his control, absent connection to desire, but it never actually became erect. The condition didn't prevent him from getting a normal erection during sex, but when his penis was not in service of our coital act, the sensation he was experiencing was very uncomfortable. And, when we did have sex, his orgasms didn't feel as robust to him. Dr. B said she'd heard that complaint in the past from men going through chemo treatments. Her recognition of the problem was unaccompanied by symptom solutions or, at minimum, connection to outside resources. I guess we just had to wait for it to subside?

When we did make love, it felt like our intimacy was infused with a deeper level of care and gentleness. We continued to crave the physical comfort we offered each other. Our silent communication took the burden of words out of the equation—offering a pipeline to exchange pure emotion. Our roles as caregiver and infirm were suspended. In bed, we remained equals—healthy lovers enjoying our decades-old relationship while appreciating our bodies born of the present moment. In this space, we felt normal.

The evening before his admittance, Jim asked me tentatively if I wanted to fool around. There was a sadness in his voice that hurt me deeply because it sounded like he was afraid my heart was leaving him. Nothing could have been further from the truth, but I could see how he might be thinking that. How could you not fear that your partner might be creating distance when you were no longer *whole* so to speak. Certainly, fear was messing with his mind. I'm sure my fear-driven behavior wasn't helping build his confidence. He reflected out loud how we hadn't had sex in a while. I'm so thankful that I eagerly took him up on his invitation. I didn't know this would be the last time our hopeful hearts and our earnest bodies would meld as one.

In the last six months of Jim's life, we created our own definition of making love. We abandoned the modern-day definition solely attributed to the physical act of sex in favor of a deeper, holistic joining that more accurately reflected our emotional experience. Our love making borrowed components from the original late 16th century definition: to pay amorous attention, to court, to woo. We were creating a new relationship out of old love. As if we were star-crossed lovers in our 20s, our world shrunk to the point where all we could see was each other. There was a tenderness in our attentions, characteristic of newlyweds.

The physical representations of our love manifested in our activities together. He cooked, did small chores and took care of little things around the house for me. We talked, walked, and enjoyed nature together. Taking care of Jim felt like a yoga practice. With gratitude, I worked in service of my husband. And he allowed me the honor of serving him unconditionally.

Buddhist monks practice generosity by accepting donations from lay people. When I first learned about their tradition of receiving, it didn't make sense to me. It sounded strange and counterintuitive. But I get it now. There's a greater opportunity to grow in relationship through the meaningful reciprocity involved in this exchange.

Over the years, my husband often rebuffed my attempts to give to him. Whether it was assistance with something or material goods like sneakers or a shirt, he'd tell me he didn't want or need what I was offering. Feeling rejected, those interactions would frustrate the heck out of me. If I'm being honest, I realize I, too, demonstrated the same behavior. We were raised to be independent in every way. Accepting someone's offers of gifts, services, or kind words was interpreted in our minds as irresponsible or weak. But our cancer experience taught us a different way of thinking. Openly receiving is a form of accepting that person. It's not about a material gain, but a knowing. A way of saying "I see you. Do you see me?" Accepting the offer creates a deeper emotional connection with the giver. That in and of itself is a gift and a generosity.

After all these years, this new perspective helped us forge a path to a greater closeness in our relationship. I cared for Jim without leveraging a power differential because I didn't perceive him as broken or *less than*. In return, Jim wholly trusted me to care for him because in this new frontier of our couplehood, we were moved to act in service of each other. Together, through giving and receiving, we discovered a new way of making love. While our minds were fully occupied with Jim's illness, over which we had so little control, our hearts were making love as we tended to each other and the familiar tasks of our small world.

CHAPTER EIGHTEEN

Paddling a Leaky Boat

The first week Jim was in the hospital, I focused on the to-do list of the treatment schedule and keeping an eye on Gianni. An uneasiness lived in my body, keeping my cortisol levels high. I told myself that Jim was undergoing so many treatments, my presence probably wouldn't be very helpful, so it was okay to sit this out.

After the first week of the transplant process, I started to enjoy the lifted responsibility of providing for Jim's care. For four months, I was his personal nurse. Driving back and forth to the infusion center, timing his medicines, keeping a close eye on his eating, sleeping and elimination habits. Being hyperaware of every single part of his daily life while plagued by never-ending worry took its toll. All the responsibilities of being his nurse were on pause for the time being, giving me some relief. That feeling didn't last long, though. First, shame showed up to scold me for enjoying the break. By the end of the second week, shame was joined by fear and anger.

I talked to Jim several times a day. We'd videochat in the morning. In the afternoon I'd drive over to the hospital and drop off packages containing a combination of cards, food, gifts from friends or clothes. Anything to inject his day with a modicum of happiness. Sometimes when he felt up to it, he'd go to his window while I stood underneath on the sidewalk. I'd call him and we'd talk—separated by six floors of concrete and glass. I couldn't really see him that well, but we still tried to be together in a reverse-Rapunzel kind of way. Those were short visits because standing at the window was uncomfortable for him, but at least they gave him a glimpse of the outside world.

Over the course of Jim's hospitalization, his condition declined. I mean, that was to be expected since the initial chemo and radiation treatments were meant to kill his bone marrow to make way for Gianni's cells. But intellectualizing the reality doesn't lift one's spirits. Chatting on the phone was a chore for him because there was nothing good to report, and he had zero interest in trying to muster false enthusiasm. He couldn't eat. There was nothing to do, no way of being comfortable or distracted. Due to Covid, he wasn't allowed to even leave his room. Physically, he felt horrible, and the living conditions had him solidly pinned down in misery.

Jim was miles away from any kind of positive attitude, and I was worried he was going to give up. The situation fanned the flames of my desperation to find ways of comforting him from afar. I persisted in sending up packages, but I don't even think he looked through them. He had zero appetite, so none of the food was touched. My notes went unacknowledged, and his cards collected in a pile on his nightstand. Still, I persisted in my daily deliveries to convey the sentiment that we were all thinking of and missing him.

Not being there in person added a different kind of stress. All I could do was ruminate on my fears. I asked the nurses to call me when the docs were on rounds. They always promised, then managed to remember maybe twice a week. Plus, even if they did call, I couldn't hear anything. Everyone was masked, and no one put any effort into making sure I could hear. Audio-visual technicians they were not. And they did not care to be.

Covid had everyone on edge, and our healthcare system—the system we rely on to be prepared for a public health crisis—seemed to be as panic-stricken as the civilians it served. With good reason. People were dying from a virus no one could explain. However, that does not give healthcare systems in the wealthiest country on the planet a pass on providing appropriate care to their non-pandemic patients. What may have seemed like common sense care for a cancer patient like Jim slowly faded. As part of his recovery, for example, Jim had to take a boatload of pills four times a day. Some of the pills were as big as quarters. A healthy person would find it exceptionally difficult to choke these bad boys down on a good day. Without thought or attention to what might make this process less hellacious, he was given the pills all at once at every dosing and expected to swallow them in one sitting. One evening, his empty stomach couldn't take it anymore. In a great big pharmacological heave, he barfed them all out. Rather than regrouping and figuring out a different approach to pill delivery, his nurse made him take them all over again. She gave no thought to modifications or even minor adjustments to make it easier for him to ingest them. When he called me to tell me about it the next morning, he was in tears. That was it. I pretty well lost my mind. I made sure Jim's morning nurse video-called me during his appointment with the attending doctor so I could give him an earful. "Is this the best you can do? Can't you stagger the pills? Cut some of the big ones in half? Create a plan that works for him if he has to take 20 pills at a time? Come on!"

During one of my video chats with Jim, I came to find out that the reason he had to cut our in-person conversations short was because he had to lean over a couch to see me on the sidewalk. A nurse helped him over to the window when I called, so they knew he was having trouble in that awkward position. Those couches were on wheels, designed to be moved for families staying over during normal times, yet no one thought to move it out of his way to make him more comfortable. Jim wasn't allowed to leave his room for fear of Covid contagion. I would think that the one visit he had with someone from the outside would be maximized in order to help his mood, possibly alleviating his stress and taking the burden of filling emotional gaps off of the nurses. I also noticed that no one had put Jim's greeting cards on the corkboard, like we did during his first hospital stay, leaving his waking eyes to fall on a blank wall instead of on festive salutations from his friends. These all sound like little things, but when you're in bad health and stuck in what feels like solitary confinement, these considerations, left unattended, contribute to a patient's negative view of their situation and their future.

To exacerbate an already troublesome situation, Jim's post BMT neuropathy worsened, dulling sensation in his extremities to such an alarming degree that he no longer had any feeling in his penis. I don't think I need to explain to most of you how devastating that is for a man. Some effects of neuropathy subside over time, but there's always the fear that they could be permanent.

My normally jovial husband was sinking fast into a depression. That's when I asked more forcefully for mental health support. A friend of mine put me in touch with a doctor in the psychiatric department who had oversight of mental health care for the cancer center. She verified that there was no permanent psychiatric staff in the cancer center, and that they were short-staffed throughout the hospital, so providing support to cancer patients was exceptionally difficult for her team. Still, she assured me she would find someone to visit Jim. One social worker visited Jim, but she went out on maternity leave shortly after that first and only meeting. His care team didn't automatically provide another mental health professional, so I had to ask *again*.

While they were scrounging the hospital for support staff, I wrote a three-page letter to the head of the cancer center to share my concerns about the glaring lack of psychosocial support for the inpatients. I followed up my letter with a phone call about a week later. When I asked to speak to the head of the cancer center by name, the person who answered the phone argued with me about who the actual head of the cancer center was. I told her I was looking at the website, and could see that the specific person I had asked for was in fact the head of the cancer center. She finally took my message.

My call was returned by our transplant nurse coordinator. I told her I wasn't calling about the transplant, and I was resolute that I wanted to talk to the head of the center about the content of my letter. I did share with her that I was concerned for Jim's mental health. I never received a follow-up call from anyone.

Eventually, another social worker showed up to talk with Jim, but at this point, it was like a firefighter showing up to a five-alarm fire with a bucket of water. There were all kinds of things wrong, but she was too late and not trained for the task at hand. The social workers in the cancer center were administrative case workers who helped patients navigate technical issues involving things like insurances and disability claims. They weren't dedicated therapists.

The person chatted politely with Jim. At the end of their conversation, he didn't see the point of meeting with her again. (Honestly, how do you tell a stranger who isn't even qualified to provide a therapeutic experience that you're afraid of dying, you feel horrid, and you can't feel your penis?) He told her he was fine and didn't need her to come back. He wasn't rejecting help, he just recognized this was not the help he needed, and this untrained stand-in was making him feel worse.

Not knowing what else to do, she handed Jim a deck of children's flashcards that count down the 100 days post-transplant, and she left. That was the fantastic patient-centered care my husband received. Doing nothing would have been less damaging, but handing him children's flash cards was an act of cruelty born of incompetence.

During my earlier call with the psychiatrist, I asked her if she had worked with the head of the cancer center to create a mental health action plan for inpatients in preparation for the Covid lockdown. She replied in the negative. I got the impression that they never spoke for the purpose of collaboration on patient care at any time, let alone in preparation for the pandemic. Both furious with our hospital and stunned by this abdication of responsibility by the head of the center, it was all I could do to keep *my* morale up while trying to support my husband from afar. What could I possibly do to help him? It felt like I was advocating for his care outside the gates of Mordor while he was on the inside dissolving in despair.

Then, during one of my frenzied cleaning jags, it hit me. A solution so simple, yet incredibly intimate and meaningful. I could read to him. Reading provided a nightly activity we could enjoy together—free from the stress of having to manufacture something to talk about. Jim could enjoy the distraction from his misery, and the closeness of my voice. And I could feel connected to him while providing the comfort and care I so desperately wanted to give him.

We both loved a good adventure, so we chose *Endurance*, the story of Lord Shackleton's harrowing voyage to Antarctica in 1914. This particular story about the 28-man crew's survival against impossible odds seemed appropriate. Every evening, as the sanguine sun claimed another minute in the sky to add to her summertime collection, I cozied into my couch and called Jim. There was no need for the perfunctory "how's it going?" We already knew. I'd wait for him to get settled, then pick up where I'd left off the night before, and together, we'd go sailing off into an hour of peace.

The caper

While Jim languished in the hospital, my mind was plagued by a parade of goblins that taunted my anxieties. I kept occupied as best I could with chores, but the room in my mind palace dedicated to worry, stress, and anxiety needed airing out. As I cleaned my house within an inch of its life, I tried to distract the residents of my worry chamber by introducing fantasies of secretly visiting Jim. At first, the scenarios I conjured acted as a pressure release valve to that intense compression chamber. But as the month lurched forward, watching Jim's condition deteriorate over video chat incited my imagination to create outlandish daydreams akin to *Mission Impossible*. I'd picture myself scaling walls, stealing nurse badges, and rappelling off the roof into open windows. My hypothetical plans started to take up an increasing amount of real estate in my psyche. As the intensity reached a fevered pitch, a more reasonable part of my brain had to intervene before I actually started acting out these scenes. Like the ghost of Christmas past, my executive function kicked open a door in my mind to screen a memory of a time when I regaled Jim with the details of an elaborate plan to break into a different public property.

The scene was Highland Park, a landscape design marvel created by Frederick Law Olmstead of Central Park fame. It boasts an intriguing collection of trees, bushes, and plants. Walking through this spectacular arrangement of nature, one can't help but be gobsmacked by Olmstead's genius. Every season sets a new stage for nature's spectacular fashion show. Even winter doesn't seem so bad when you wind your way around the sleeping magnolias and lilac bushes. It's absolutely magical.

There's a small greenhouse tucked away in the middle of the park. This little gem is home to a tight collection of domestic and exotic plants. Some of the cacti and palms are upwards of 14' tall. They smoosh into the top of the greenhouse while flowering vines wind around them to create a rain forest-like canopy. Turtles rule the water features while tortoises keep watch over the desert plants like praetorian guards. It only takes five minutes to walk through. But if you care to linger, it's easy to imagine that you're miles away from civilization.

In December, the conservatory is adorned with multicolored lights. As winter darkness settles in disturbingly early, the soft glow from the decorations provides just enough light to mark your way. I love to sit on a camouflaged bench in quiet reverence. This winter oasis makes up the backdrop for one of my last memories of a healthy, happy Jim. I'd wanted to enjoy the garden lights with Jim for years, but their limited hours didn't fit into his schedule. It just so happened that, on this particular night, while on our evening walk, we discovered that the greenhouse had extended their hours. I was thrilled! We finally got to enjoy the holiday lights together.

We ambled through, admiring the myriad varieties of poinsettias and Christmas cacti. Eventually, we came to the center of the garden and decided to sit a while. We talked in hushed tones while listening to the water trickling from the fountains around us. The warm, humid air had a soporific effect, lulling us into silent contemplation.

After sitting in silence for some time, I interrupted our reverie with the pronouncement that I wanted to spend the night there. Shocked and intrigued, Jim asked how I was going to pull off this ridiculous caper. A back and forth ensued as I wove an elaborate plan to elude the caretakers, find a comfortable place to sleep, and exit the next morning undetected. He was not as convinced as I was of the failsafe nature of my plan. After brief consideration, he announced that he would not be joining me. But he offered to sleep with his phone on in case I needed assistance...or bail.

Eventually, all tuckered out from spinning my yarn, I quieted down and we continued to enjoy each other's company in what felt like our own private sanctuary. At closing time, we dutifully exited into the street lit night. The neighborhood decorations were bright and cheery, welcoming us back to the cold crisp air. Spiritually sated by our commune with nature, we walked the last mile home, gloved hand in gloved hand.

The workings of the human brain are a wonder. In my time of extreme duress, my brain recalled this memory to pacify my obsession with sneaking into the hospital and left me soothed enough to focus on the reality around me and get through another day.

The ants go marching in

Though my psyche found a coping corner, the physical manifestation of my agitation needed to be engaged continuously. As June wore on, regular chores and exercise were proving to be insufficient occupations. I needed more. It may sound awful, but I suppose what happened next actually helped me by providing an outsized task to focus on. Afterall, what better distraction is there than uninvited house guests?

One morning, I woke up and started my daily routine per usual. When I entered my kitchen to make coffee, I was startled to see my ants had arrived for their annual visit. This was unexpected—with everything going on I never factored in that this might be an actual thing that didn't go away because—well, because I had bigger things to worry about. Even more upsetting was the fact that this particular year they brought their friends. Thousands of them.

Unlike human aunts, there are no casseroles or cookies in the offing. No, these little suckers expect to be *served*. There they were, hanging out around my kitchen sink like spring breakers in Daytona. They acted so casual, as if I would be happy to welcome them back. I went out back to discover that there was an offensive being staged by multiple colonies.

Enraged at the audacity of these interlopers, I suited up like Rambo, and with all my jumpy energy, I waged a scorched earth campaign to rid my domain of the ant battalions. Like a general overlooking a battlefield map, I strategically planned the placement of diatomaceous earth and borax bombs. Once I had my plans solidified, I got to work mixing my concoctions in preparation for war.

Concurrent to waging war on the ant colonies, I approached gardening with intensity and fervor. I was a woman possessed, swinging from exacting death and destruction one minute to creating life the next. Ant colonies were beaten back with daily bombings and yard reformations while my pampered pumpkin patch and heirloom tomatoes were growing as aggressively as Jack's beanstalk. In hindsight, I wonder if I was subconsciously acting out the battle happening inside Jim's body?

If so, I wasn't the only one. The pandemic was now fully raging through the world. Finger-pointing and mixed messaging plastered the news. Global leaders were trying desperately to keep fear and panic from driving the bus, while people were dying all around us. We witnessed both heroic acts of selflessness by healthcare providers and the basest of selfishness by people getting into fistfights over the merits of wearing small rectangles of cotton on their faces. People's nerves were stretched past capacity. Then, when you thought things couldn't get any worse, George Floyd was murdered. Publicly. In broad daylight. By someone paid to serve and protect.

Protests and demonstrations erupted across the nation— some transforming into violence at sunset. Bite-sized Rochester experienced a major metropolitan response, joining the Black Lives Matter movement with full-throated solidarity. Business owners in my neighborhood boarded up their windows in a flash. My vibrant community of 30 years looked like a war zone.

Giacomo and Gianni joined the rallies and protests with friends. I was proud of them, but at the same time, it created a whole new category of worry. The rallies meant high Covid exposures and, at times, spikes of violence. Tensions were high. It was all too much. As a nation, we were already losing our minds, but after the tragedy of George Floyd's murder, we just about lost our faith.

CHAPTER NINETEEM

Shock and Awe

Day 30 of the transplant calendar was the target date for Jim's discharge, but the possibility that he wouldn't be strong enough to come home then was fast becoming a probability. Before I could dissolve into total despair over a potential hospitalization extension, I got some good news. Jim reported that the nurses wanted me to come in for a "teach-in" to show me how to administer medicines and change his IV when he came home.

I was ecstatic! I felt like oxygen hit my lungs for the first time in 30 days. I dutifully got my Covid test and prepared to see my husband. On June eighth, I crossed the Covid moat and went up to Jim's floor with "first-day-of-school" butterflies.

When I arrived, the center was unrecognizable. Chairs and tables in common areas had been removed. Signs and tape directing people's movements adorned the hall walls and floors. The hustle bustle was replaced by an eerie quiet. What was most distressing was the family waiting area. When I got off the elevator and turned the corner, I walked into emptiness. Yes, a physical emptiness, but what was more disquieting was the absence of the family spirit. The collective of life's energy

I previously described had been scrubbed out of the area as thoroughly as I had exterminated ants from my house. From this description, you might expect it felt mournful, which is what I would have preferred over what I was met with. This existential vibey place had become the harbor for all the fear and anxiety that was leaking from the healthcare staff.

It was here, in this stark white hallway, that I received a battery of instructions on how to care for my husband. They told me all about the million medicines, about IV care and what graft versus host disease would look like, should we suffer that on top of all the other side effects of this treatment phase. But they didn't prepare me for what I was about to receive. Here, in this cold space devoid of any human joy, they wheeled out Jim. To my horror, the waiting area wasn't the only thing that was unrecognizable.

It's criminal what our society does to people under the guise of *healthcare*. It's an even higher crime that the cancer complex is a multi-billion-dollar industry that has made a disgusting number of people wealthy. Health insurers, hospitals, pharmaceutical companies...cancer is their milk cow that produces in perpetuity. The perfunctory effort put into actually stopping the causes of cancer pales in comparison. We have been polluting our environment with carcinogens and toxic chemicals for decades in the name of capitalism, or progress, or whatever you want to call it. And we stand for it! People spray their yards with Roundup, while our women battle breast cancer. We suck on vapes while an alarming number of people whither from lung cancer. And we drink water—of all things—out of plastic bottles while our children are afflicted with blood cancers. Yet all we can do is write a check, or run in a 5k, thinking that's helping to solve the problem and content ourselves with the pretense that cancer is "the luck of the draw." It's absolute bullshit.

When I laid eyes on my husband for the first time since his transplant, my heart stopped. My eyes begged my brain to understand that the image being delivered was true and real. It's like my eyes had to grab my brain by the lapels and shake it yelling: "Wake Up! We need you! NOW!" My brain came to fast enough to stop the chest-welling shriek of "WHAT HAVE YOU DONE TO MY HUSBAND?!"

The nurses were nervously twittering around like Disney characters on meth as they tried to infuse the air with excitement over our "reunion." Meanwhile, I was trying to reconcile my feelings of elation and horror. My strong, healthy husband who had been my protector and provider throughout our life together, the man who had the strength and spirit of a warrior, now looked like a POW being released from a gulag.

Jim appeared sickly, shaking and so thin his clothes were hanging off of him. Most of his face was hidden by a big black helmet and a mask. All I could see of his face were two sunken eyes peering out from dark circles. Those beautiful brown eyes twinkled with love and relief at seeing me in person. Despite my shock, I know my eyes twinkled right back at him.

The nurses continued to buzz with their "Everything's fine! Everything's fine!" cheery vibes in their attempt to coax a celebratory moment. Their false enthusiasm reminded me of parents trying to convince their three-year-old that getting a cavity filled is going to be fun. I thought: *What is wrong with all of you?! Hasn't cancer brutalized and humiliated us enough? Get away from us. You don't get to be part of our intimacy.* I tried to block them out as we cried and hugged. We were so relieved to be together again. Later on, one nurse went so far as to complain that she hadn't been able to be there for our reunion moment. I found her assumption that she was welcome into our relationship repugnant.

The physical therapist presented herself and quickly taught me how to walk with Jim using the gait belt and walker. She demonstrated on Jim, then had me practice. Stunned by the fact that Jim wasn't able to walk, I did my best to focus on learning the process. She rushed through her instructions so fast; I wondered if she was afraid of catching Covid or if she was wanting to escape before my "What the fuck is happening with my husband?" mind actually caught up.

Once the training was complete, we said our hopeful goodbyes. I watched as they wheeled Jim back to the ward, encouraged by the promise of his release in 3 days. While I made my way home, trying to digest what was going on, my shock slowly transitioned to awe. The initial shriek that got caught in my chest was now a mournful "what have you done to my husband?" whisper in my heart.

When I got home, I snapped into project management mode, coordinating all the necessary tasks in preparation for Jim's homecoming. I coordinated the runs to the hospital pharmacy, family Covid tests, deliveries of IV materials, and made preliminary introductions and tentative appointments with the physical therapists and home nurses.

The cancer center didn't send an occupational therapist to our house in advance to show me what adaptations I would need to support Jim in his weakened state. Again, not knowing what I didn't know, I never thought to ask. But the night before Jim came home, it started to dawn on me that our house, built in 1920, might need some modification. The first clue hit me like a lightning bolt while I stood in my front hall running through my mental checklist. I was about to take the stairs when my eyes scanned upward. The subconscious command to move forward slowly bloomed into a conscious thought as I rose up one stair to the next: *The stairs. The* **stairs***. Oh My God! THE STAIRS!* We didn't have a railing in our stairwell. There are 16 stairs total. Eleven stairs ascend to a landing. Once there, you have to make a 180-degree turn to tackle the remaining five. Our second floor is where both our bedroom and bathroom are. And Jim could barely stand let alone walk. I called Giacomo in a panic and tried to cajole him into installing a railing. He said "Mom, even if I YouTube it, I'm gonna make a mess. I can't do it. You need to call Kurt."

Jim did most of the work on our house, but occasionally, he would need a hand. In those instances, there was a short list of people that had the *"Jim Barbero Seal of Approval."* Those folks were either family members or lifelong friends. There was but one outsider on the list, and that was Kurt, the handy-dandy handyman.

Kurt stands about 6'4" and is as thin as a reed. When he walks, his willowy frame creates the illusion that he's actually gliding. He has a laid-back demeanor, sort of hippy-ish, but with much more purpose and resolve. His accent, a mish-mosh of southern drawl and New York hillbilly, gives away his country address. Kurt's physique belies his remarkable strength, which is often demonstrated by the requirements of a particular job. I've watched him single-handedly move, lift and demolish concrete stairs, cast iron tubs, and tree trunks the size of small cars.

Jim met Kurt while he was working on a friend's house years ago. His handiwork was excellent, but it was his sense of humor and grounded nature that attracted Jim. Plus, both men inherited a blue collar, Depression-era work ethic, so there was an automatic understanding between them about how stuff got done.

I was afraid Kurt wouldn't be available on such short notice, but necessity dictated that I give him a call. When I got his voicemail, I resigned myself to the fact that the railing wouldn't be installed in time, so I started racking my brain for a Plan B. Much to my great relief, Kurt returned my call before I pretzeled my mind to invent unworkable solutions. Kurt listened thoughtfully while I explained our dilemma. He said he could do it for me the next morning and gave me a materials shopping list for Giacomo. Like clockwork, Kurt showed up and in no time, we had a sturdy railing in our stairwell. I tried to pay him, but he refused compensation.

Our shared humanity creates a bridge for caring, kindness and compassion to spread if we let it. In the midst of my panic, Kurt did more for me than install a railing free of charge. His selflessness reminded me that I wasn't alone and that the fellowship of man would lift me up and fortify my courage to face the daunting task ahead.

On a hot summer night

According to the National Institutes of Health, the risk of life-threatening reactions to a bone marrow transplant are highest during the first 100 days post-procedure. If you make it without any major incidents, you're out of the darkest part of the woods. In those first 50 days that goalpost seemed light-years away. Second by second, our family crawled toward the 100-day mark, dragging hope behind us.

Thinking back to the offers we received from friends to connect Jim with transplant survivors, I realize now that the experiences relayed would've been influenced by a positive bias. It makes sense that survivor hindsight is heavily edited by the protective cover of selective memory, much like that of a new mother. "How was your two-day labor that ended in C-section?" "Oh, it wasn't that bad. I'm ready for another baby." Unlike new moms, BMT survivors don't ever have an urge to go through it again. The similarity lies in the fact that they've likely blocked out the gory details to enjoy the reward of cure and a subsequent feeling of gratitude. For obvious reasons, the people who didn't make it to day 100 weren't around to tell us about their experiences. But I bore witness, so I can tell you that it's so awful I can't believe it's legal.

When I picked Jim up from the hospital, his condition was shocking. Driving home on high alert with a carload of medical equipment, medicines and instructions instilled the same precarious feeling I had when we brought our first son home, but without the excitement of possibility. Technically, Jim *was* in the process of being born again. The chemotherapies and radiation treatments physically reduced Jim's body to a freakish infancy. Regenerating a healthy man was a heavy lift for Gianni's transfused blood cells. The physical agony resulting from the procedure engulfed Jim. He was suffering the depths of misery brought on by the gamble we made to pursue *cure*. Here we all were acting like Prometheus overstepping our mortal bounds to play God. It seemed reincarnation was the punishment itself. There was no need for an eagle to peck at our livers in perpetuity.

We created a care station in the living room to try and make him as comfortable as possible. Exhausted and freezing, he slept swaddled in a pile of blankets on our living room couch while I micro-assessed his needs. In the first couple of weeks, we only moved him upstairs at night so he could enjoy the comfort of our bed. Though it was an unseasonably warm June, the electric blanket was cranked to keep him warm. You could've hatched chickens in our bedroom. As a menopausal woman it felt like we were sleeping in hell.

Helping Jim walk was harrowing. His legs were like cooked spaghetti with water balloons in place of feet. Due to the neuropathy, he didn't know where his legs were in space, which made him incredibly wobbly. Thus, the necessity of a walker with physical assist. His tailor-made helmet was a mandatory accessory for the few times he ventured off the couch. Without it, a blow to the head from a fall could be lethal.

Navigating the stairs was a family effort. In the morning I'd assist Jim by holding his Gait belt as instructed while he used his walker to shuffle from our bedroom to the top of the stairs. Once he grabbed on to the banister, Gianni would run the walker down to the landing, next to a relief chair. Though it was only five stairs, by the time we got there, Jim would need a rest. Giacomo held Jim by the belt from behind while I stood in front of them, one step down. With all three of us working together, we'd walk slowly, stair step by stair step, to the landing. Jim would steady himself on the walker and shuffle over to the chair for a break. Once he was ready to tackle the rest of the stairs, Gianni would take the walker down to the main floor while Jim, Giacomo and I worked the same system down the remaining stairs. The previous year, we had spent an entire week hiking countless miles through the mountains of Wyoming. Not 10 months later, Jim could barely walk 10 steps from the living room to the dining room.

The pharmaceutical regimen was astounding. At seven columns across and four rows down, the daily pill organizer was as big as my notebook. An unbelievable number of pills were prescribed to be taken four times a day to fend off graft versus host disease, protect his vital organs, and generally prop Jim up so the regeneration process could work. The pills varied in sizes. Some were as small as a little button, while others were as large as a quarter. They gave me a pill cutter, but for the larger pills eligible for splitting, I needed our Sawzall. I could understand why he was throwing them up in the hospital. Choking all those pills down was tough. Nausea and general malaise made Jim gag at the thought of ingesting anything. But the daily pill cocktails were required, as was getting enough liquid in him, so we had to be strategic and flexible. Staggering his morning pills over the course of an hour, for example, seemed to help Jim keep them down. But new issues constantly emerged, requiring different solutions. I learned that Jim would automatically vomit first thing in the morning if I gave him the pills before he went to the bathroom. And, he'd vomit if he drank what his stomach considered to be too much water before he took his pills. His stomach constantly changed its mind over these things, so trying to plan around it was crazy-making.

While working to manage all Jim's care needs, other ailments presented themselves, exacerbating his discomfort. For Father's Day, he received an itchy rash that spread all over his head, face, and neck. Then thrush bloomed in his mouth. The accompanying remedies added more complications to the daily medicinal regimen. He wasn't supposed to drink anything a half hour before or after he used the prescription mouth rinse—which was four times a day. Wanting to avoid adding yet another oral medicine to his pill diet, I tried three topical creams to sooth his rash. None of them worked so I relented in favor of an oral Benadryl. Honestly, I felt like one of those street musicians that had a base drum strapped to my stomach, a harmonica around my neck, cymbals between my knees, and a squeeze box in my hands. During my act, the audience threw things at me to juggle while I played requests.

For the first seven days post-discharge, Jim had to go to the hospital for transfusions. Getting him up, dressed, toileted, plied with the first round of pills, down the stairs and into the car felt like a decathlon. Once he was safely delivered to the outpatient center, I'd go home and sterilize everything in the house, get reorganized and order any other supplies we needed before picking him up for round two.

Though it was a lot to manage, being the ringmaster of the daily cancer carnival didn't bother me nearly as much as his lack of appetite and food refusal. Never in my 30 years with Jim Barbero had I ever seen him turn down food of any kind. Not only was it disturbing to see him emaciated, but it was emotionally distressing to know that he was so sick he wouldn't even consider eating. And I don't mean cheeseburgers. I mean a half a teaspoon of Jell-O, or pudding, or Ensure, or ANYTHING. I thought for sure if he just had a tiny bit of something, he would feel a slight bit better. This was the issue that made my heart retreat to a corner and sit hugging its knees to rock with worry.

Assisting Jim with his ablutions was another major event in the recuperation decathlon. Our narrow bathroom had needed updating since the day we moved in, but it never made Jim's construction list. I not-so-lovingly refer to it as the "indoor outhouse." A clawfoot tub and toilet take up the left wall. The sink faces the toilet not two feet away on the right wall. Moving

Jim into the bathroom with his walker was a tight squeeze. There wasn't enough room for me to hold on to him once he got between the sink and the toilet, so I stood by nervously while he slowly turned the walker and his body inch by inch, until he made the quarter turn and was in position to sit down. I helped him with his pants, then held on to him to guide him onto the toilet seat, which all of a sudden seemed like a far drop into a gully. Trying to juggle among the walker, the sink, and holding Jim didn't go well the first time. He landed hard on the seat, resulting in an unbelievably large bruise—evidencing the state of his blood counts. I felt horrible and jumped immediately into self-attack mode for not being more careful.

Almost two weeks after Jim's discharge, an occupational therapist finally came over to help me with home adaptations. She walked me through the house, room by room, sharing tips and tricks. She was the one who told me about toilet seat extenders (who knew there was such a thing?), how to set a bench in the tub, and the best way to shower Jim. Not only was it a relief to have the knowledge, but she gave me a little more confidence in what I was doing.

Every single day was packed with Jim's care needs. As we worked on it all together, Jim became increasingly despondent. The activities that would normally help him cope were either eliminated or strictly limited by his condition. Neuropathy was a big culprit for many barriers to previously enjoyed activities. He couldn't feel his hands, so he couldn't sketch or paint, text his friends or play any instruments. With Covid raging through the world, we certainly couldn't have any visitors. Phone calls, the "light" version of human interaction, were limited because he felt so shitty and tired. All he could really do was sleep or watch television, with the latter being profoundly depressing for an active person who doesn't typically watch TV.

Discouraged by his perceived lack of progress, Jim started canceling his physical and occupational therapy appointments. When I found out he was canceling, I gently coaxed him into reconsidering. I'd extol the virtues of having the professionals come to work his muscles, chat with him and check his progress. Too tired to argue with me, he'd relent and let me reschedule the appointments.

Throughout these difficult days, it felt like I was clinging to a buoy in an angry sea gripping Jim's wrist and begging him to hold on. There were moments when I could feel him letting go, but I wouldn't have it. I bulldozed my way through like the stubborn Polack I am. Despite his emphatic protestations, I picked up a used recumbent bike and bought him a new pair of sneakers. (Initially, he couldn't wear shoes because his feet were so swollen.) Though he didn't say it, I think he was afraid he would never get to the point where he could use those things and having them around represented false hope. I was holding up optimism for both of us that his condition would improve and I wanted to be ready to get him moving as soon as it seemed feasible. Even if that meant putting on sneakers as one goal, and merely sitting on the bike another. Those activities would be enough proof of progress to convince *hope* that it was welcome to take a seat in our house.

All of our "one step forward, two steps back" efforts were draining me physically and emotionally. One day, I sat in my office and just stared out the window. Though it was a beautiful summer day, there seemed to be a thin gray veil dulling its vibrancy. I remember thinking: "There must be a better way to do this." We needed help, but I was stymied. Stymied by Covid.

Stymied by our healthcare system. Stymied by the many-tentacled beast that was cancer choking every single aspect of our lives. My mournful reflections were interrupted by a phone call. It was my old college roommate Molly. Though we didn't talk often, I held her in my heart as one of my dearest friends. Molly is an elementary school principal who is kind, compassionate, fiercely intelligent, and selfless. A perfect combination of character traits for someone overseeing the education of little ones. Molly's dedication to her school and her kids is legend in Western New York. Relieved to hear her voice, I shared with her the challenges we were facing. Molly listened intently, then, after a thoughtful pause, said, "Well, you know my brother Dennis is an oncology social worker at Kaiser Permanente in Denver. I bet he'd be happy to talk to Jim. I'll text him right now and send you his number." And just like that, the veil was lifted.

It's amazing how precious gifts were delivered every time I was stuck on *What do we do now?* moments. Dennis had decades of experience providing psychotherapeutic support to his oncology patients, and he had the added benefit of being male and a contemporary of Jim's. I reached out to Dennis immediately. We had a great conversation. He completely understood everything we were going through and without hesitation offered to talk to Jim. For the first time my feelings of fear, loss, and concern for Jim's mental health during his recovery were being validated. I was nervous about approaching Jim with the invitation to talk with Dennis. If he passed up the opportunity, I knew it meant we were at rock bottom. Although Jim had never met Dennis before, he loved and trusted Molly. In his mind, it would follow suit that any brother of Molly's must be pretty special. To my great relief, Jim enthusiastically accepted the idea.

After connecting them, I got out of the way so Jim could feel free to talk about everything that was on his mind and in his heart. They talked for an hour straight. When they hung up, I could see relief on Jim's face and a spark of life restored in his eyes. That's the kicker. It didn't take much—just someone to understand, to see Jim as a person and to let him know that he mattered. It was incredibly validating for my husband. They agreed to keep talking on a regular basis.

Around the same time Jim spoke with Dennis, he seemed to be making tiny physical improvements. He started to take an interest in doing his physical therapy exercises. He ordered hand therapy balls and wanted to sit on the porch in the sun for part of the day. Not long after, he asked the boys to help him put his sneakers on and assist him onto the recumbent bike so he could get a feel for it. Were we truly turning a corner?!

On day 41, we received the amazing news that the cancer cells were undetectable in Jim's bloodwork. Gianni's cells were performing the intended curative work! Reaching this milestone was cause for celebration, carrying with it the reward of ditching the helmet! We actually started to feel like we were on the right side of the 50/50 coin toss.

As the next week went by, things really started looking up. We saw more improvements in Jim's strength. He was showing interest in food and taking charge of his exercises. The medicine schedule remained rigorous, the home visits from his care team continued to be a regular part of Jim's routine, and he still had to go to the hospital for appointments, but he was starting to smile. In the late mornings, I would set him up on our porch to enjoy the weather. He'd have his water with electrolyte drops on the table beside him, next to a dish of my latest attempt to feed him, his IV pole with a tube plugged into his port, and a floppy hat to keep the sun off his skin. It was an ordeal, but worth the effort to see him exhibit a desire to do something, even if it was just sitting on the porch. Our sons would sit out there with him, chitchatting and joking together. A couple of friends here and there would come by for brief lawn visits, taking great care to sit as far away as their voices would carry. Jim got tired quickly and napped often, but he was visibly cultivating purpose. He even ate a small plate of Chinese food for dinner that week. That action alone lifted a weight of worry off my mind.

Wanting to capitalize on Jim's progress, I started taking him on mini fieldtrips to practice walking in different spots around our neighborhood. We'd walk about 10 steps with his walker, then turn around and walk back to the car and sit awhile in our camp chairs like tailgaters. We'd chat a bit or sit in silence breathing the fresh air, giving Jim time to muster up the energy to get back in the car to go home.

Jim's returning strength was accompanied by a smattering of optimism. He had the idea to go shopping for a left-handed electric guitar—wanting to use it as a training tool to get his hands back in shape. Watching him look at guitars made me giddy. He hemmed and hawed about spending the money. It was so good to see his frugality on full display, like he was getting back to his old self. I actually had to talk him into buying the guitar: "Honey! You've been through hell! You deserve to buy yourself a good present!" After playing with a few guitars, he picked out a gorgeous Fender Stratocaster and was as excited to bring it home as a kid at Christmas.

The fourth of July was Jim's day 50—the halfway point. That week, we celebrated a different kind of "Independence Day" when Jim graduated from using the walker to walking with a cane, and put himself on a low-key fitness routine. Day 100 was glowing a little brighter at the end of our tunnel as *hope* got out of its chair in the corner and started to move among us.

The following week, while we were enjoying the latest progress in Jim's recovery, something strange happened in our house. Gianni came up from the basement and announced that there was a housefly infestation in the basement bathroom. Not the whole basement, just the bathroom, even though the door was open. I went to see for myself and sure enough, a swarm of houseflies was buzzing around, self-containing in the bathroom. I'd never seen anything like it. We looked everywhere and couldn't find the source. It was as disgusting as it was inexplicable. Something about the infestation had an ominous, Old Testament quality to it.

CHAPTER TWENTY

Déjà Vu

We were a solid week past the midpoint when Jim experienced a night of restlessness. Discomfort stopped being remarkable months ago, so it wasn't cause for alarm. Besides, we were all enjoying Jim's progress as he continued to make noticeable improvements. In the morning, I dropped him off at the cancer center per usual so he could get pumped up with whatever his labs of the day deemed necessary. He was already scheduled to meet with his transplant doctor after his transfusion, so he was prepared to talk about his difficult night at his appointment. I was busy with chores around the house while waiting for the phone call to include me in the conversation with his doctor.

The phone chimed right on time. My unsuspecting mind anticipated the barrage of medical jargon from Jim's doctor before I was given the okay to come pick him up. Jim's voice greeted me with the two words I miss the most. "Hi honey." Then, without any pause or preamble he said: "The leukemia is back." He didn't sound alarmed, nor did he sound relaxed. There was a wonder in his voice as if he was standing in the path of a tsunami, knowing there was nowhere to go, no way to protect himself and no time to react. This was his time. Now.

Giacomo was milling about when I let out a gasp. He looked at me in alarm, and I scribbled "Leukemia is back." on my notebook. His face went blank as he stared at the words on the page. Jim then switched his phone to speaker so I could hear the transplant doctor go over his blood test results. My brain was hanging on his every word, waiting to hear that we could still win this fight. He'd ordered a biopsy to check if it truly was a relapse. The doctor wanted to readmit Jim to the cancer center while he waited for the biopsy results and assessed other options. Thankfully, I was given permission to enter the hospital and join Jim in his room.

When I arrived, the doctor came in again to talk with both of us. I could see he was crestfallen. It was clear he didn't want this new development to be true. Sincerely and without ego, he did not want Jim to die. This wasn't about physician failure; this was about being human. I was touched by his caring reaction.

For 48 hours we held our breaths, waiting to get the biopsy results and learn about possible treatment options. The results verified what we suspected. The cancer was back. Jim was so weak and sickly from the BMT, it would be inhumane to subject him to anymore treatments. This death knell sent ice through my veins. Everything my husband suffered was for naught. Caught in the clutches of cancer and the pandemic, these evil twins were incessantly dealing blows to one so undeserving of this agony. The cruelty of it all was incomprehensible.

Despite the biopsy results, Jim's team wanted to make sure all options were thoroughly vetted. We were in a hospital after all, so a bunch more doctors' tickets needed to get punched for billing purposes. In hindsight, this was the time we should have been supported in a nesting process to prepare for Jim's passing.

A new merry-go-round of medical teams came through. If I wasn't comfortable with it at the beginning, I certainly had had enough of this parade of the absurd now. Cardiology was called to run some tests. A student-led team of five people swooped in like death vultures, eager to view what they'd only read about in textbooks. A while back, a lawyer friend of mine had told me that I had the right to refuse people in our hospital room. With that in mind, I told the resident leading the cardiology team that I only wanted necessary personnel in the room. For Christ's sake, we just learned my husband's cancer was back. Jim didn't need the added humiliation of being viewed like a sideshow freak. With all the emotional intelligence of a three-year-old, the young doctor pushed back with a snotty and aggressive "Everyone on my team is necessary." Without skipping a beat, my eyes flicked to the only person in the crowd who had gray hair. I deduced that he was the attending responsible for the resident. He was staring hard at the floor, avoiding my gaze as if the exchange would go unnoticed if he didn't look up. I ignored the resident and addressed the older doctor, releasing each word in a short burst like they were rocks I was whipping at his head: "Only. Who. Is. Necessary." The doctor nodded slightly without looking at me and excused the superfluous three. The resident and the attending proceeded to examine Jim and, well, stuff was going down with Jim's cardiopulmonary system. That's about all I can say, because at that point, everything I heard was muffled like I was under water.

By Wednesday, July 15, the reality we knew deep down was now being verbalized by the healthcare team: there were no more practical treatment options. Our fate had been determined. The person who came in to convey this news was the doctor I'd yelled at after Jim threw up on his pills in the first week post-transplant. I was comfortable with him because during that previous incident, he demonstrated his ability to tolerate my anger and acted accordingly by adjusting Jim's care. His plain, honest, commonsense words and actions won me over. He had an ego air about him, but it seemed his ego could make room for mine in a way that allowed for open communication. He told us that Jim had a week or two left. Maybe more. The "maybe more" was almost like a disclaimer because you never know *exactly* when someone will die, but the emphasis on: "within a week or two" was loud and clear.

Exhaustion, fear, and sadness weighed us down. All we wanted to do was go home, but before we could leave, we had to meet with the palliative team to make more care decisions. The doctor assigned to us was clearly well regarded because his arrival was preceded by much fanfare from our healthcare staff. I wonder if it was nervous energy that bumped up their exuberance, because their excitement around telling us how wonderful the palliative care doctor was bordered on the fanatical. "Oh, you're going to see Dr. Wonderful! He's so great! You're going to like him. He was one kind of doctor, then went back to medical school to become a palliative doctor because he liked the discipline so much and blah blah blah, wonderful wonderful wonderful, blah blah blah."

I'm always suspect when someone gets rave reviews. Once that "wonderful" word starts rolling off peoples' tongues, any bystander with a negative view is more inclined to keep it to themselves so as not to be in the "out crowd." Let's face it, "wonderful" is not only subjective, but it's a high bar. The "He's so wonderful!" groupthink controls critique and subdues curiosity to explore other possibilities. Basically, it's a social belt sander for rough spots.

The doctor sent in to talk to us about palliative and hospice care didn't provide any useful information for me to take home. For example, he did not tell me what a body goes through when it dies. He did not explain how to take Jim off his current medications, while introducing the new medications being prescribed, or what the possible effects of changing all his medications would have on him. He didn't tell me how to make Jim comfortable or how to deal with any pain Jim may experience. In a nutshell, he didn't tell me anything generally about how to care for someone who is actively dying or specifically about how to help my husband die with dignity. He may have been smart. He may have been a good guy. However, he was automatically disqualified from the wonderful category because as an end-of-life healthcare professional, he neglected to talk about death and dying to his dying patient and that patient's caregiver.

Essentially, Dr. Wonderful gave us a didactic presentation on the differences between palliative and hospice care. He was spewing an administrative tangle of words developed by health insurance companies to categorize care for billing purposes. There I sat heartbroken and in shock, trying to glean from his dissertation anything that would help me care for my husband in his final days, while white noise poured out of his mouth in an unrelenting stream. I suspected there was more information I needed. Much more. But, for the umpteenth time, I was stuck in that void of not knowing what I didn't know, so the right questions eluded me.

Finally, I gave up trying to understand. Jim was getting increasingly impatient—rightfully so—and just wanted to go home. The doctor's presentation ended with "Do you want palliative care or hospice care?" From an elementary perspective, it sounded like Jim would get more care as a palliative patient than with hospice, so that's what we chose. Since Jim's passing, I found out that most medical professionals can't effectively explain the difference between palliative and hospice care. Unless you're an end-of-life care provider, the line between the two is blurry, so I'll do my best to give you a quick overview.

Palliative care is covered by your regular health insurance (that is, if you have health insurance) and provides for both comfort care (which includes pain relief and symptom management), *and* curative care for a serious illness or disease. Hospice care is funded by Medicare and only covers comfort care at end-of-life. The important difference is that if you are prescribed palliative care, your health insurance will continue to cover curative treatment for all your health care issues, not just the ones presenting from your terminal illness. For example, if you have chronic obstructive pulmonary disease (COPD) and depression, in addition to a terminal cancer diagnosis, under palliative care, treatment for all your diagnoses will continue to be covered. If you go into hospice care, Medicare won't cover any life-extending medicines for your cancer. You would rely on your regular health coverage to continue to treat your COPD and depression (again, if you have other health insurance). But it isn't a foregone conclusion that your health insurer would approve your treatment for your other healthcare needs. A big problem arises when those needs are subject to the interpretation of the patient's provider and their health insurer. Using the same example, if you opt for hospice care because of your cancer and suffer complications from your COPD, you may have to fight with your provider to pay for your prescriptions because they may categorize *any* treatment as "life-extending."

That's one of the issues with a profit-driven healthcare system. Many hospice patients are in good shape for several months and can enjoy a decent quality of life until they pass if they have the right medical support. But whether or not you are able to comfortably maximize what little time you have left depends on your health insurance coverage.

Another important aspect of end-of-life care that I learned only after volunteering in hospice for a year is that if you take your loved one home to die, you don't receive daily nursing support. Both with Jim and with my father, I expected a team of hospice angels to descend on my home and to help us manage the complicated and difficult stages of dying. That was a big part of the problem of not having anything properly explained to us. My expectations for care were high, only to be met by the reality of a system that doesn't value patients they can no longer bill. The only way you get daily nursing support at home is if you private pay a lot of money. And that's in non-pandemic times. During the pandemic, homecare nurses and certified nursing assistants were scarce. In non-pandemic times, if you aren't private paying for assistance, once you transition to home hospice, a car drives by and a nurse throws a brown paper bag full of morphine out their window as they speed by your house. Of course, I'm exaggerating. But not by much. Here in New York, you get a home visit from a nurse for an hour at most, once or twice a week. If you really press the staffing agency, you might be able to get a certified nursing assistant (if any are available) to help with your loved one's personal care twice a week for a couple hours. All other care is provided by the patient's family or chosen caregiver. That's 24/7 personal hygiene, feeding, toileting, bed changing, laundry, administering medicines, and, of course, worrying.

If you have insurance and want round-the-clock care, your best option is to enter a healthcare facility like a hospital, nursing home, or hospice house. Those institutions have the equipment and trained staff to provide the type of hands-on care and real-time assessments to keep your loved one as comfortable as possible. But where you can receive care and the quality of that care always depends on what kind of insurance you have and room availability.

Many of us speculate on how we want to die from time to time, but where one wants to die is a decision that requires much more than speculation. Having gone through it twice, I highly recommend you add it to your list of "important topics for discussion" with your family if you want to avoid traumatizing yourself and your loved ones. That's why you should be having that discussion with your family and friends before you actually need it. Because trying to make that decision while under extreme duress is a nightmare.

As we were going through the discharge process, there was one nurse (of course it was a nurse) who gently shared with us what people in her life did when they knew they were going to die. Things like giving special items to certain people or making a photobook of memories. Mostly, she talked to us about making the most of our time together as Jim was coming to the final days of his life. Those were words we could hear and understand. And those were the words Jim let guide him as he planned out his final days.

On Friday, July 17, I brought Jim home to die. We left the hospital with the promise that a palliative nurse was going to see us on Saturday. Wading deeper into the unknown, I held my breath and braced myself to manage whatever was going to come our way .

When we got home, I made Jim comfortable in his living room station. The place where he'd been in various stages of illness for months, surrounded by his sketchpads, instruments and cats, was now the place he would nest in preparation for his passing. As Jim sunk into the couch resigned, Giacomo and Gianni sat next to each other on the loveseat opposite him. The three of us didn't know what to do or say. But Jim did. He told his sons how proud he was of them—that they'd become fine young men, and he loved them very much. Then he broke down and cried. The boys sat in silence, wide-eyed and numb as reality wrung their souls out like dishrags. Their hero. Their best friend. Their Dad. After fighting so hard. After suffering sickness, pain, and unending indignities, much of which was suffered in trying to stay with them. Their Dad was about to leave them forever. How could that be?

> "And you, my father, there on the sad height, Curse, bless, me now with your fierce tears, I pray. Do not go gentle into that good night. Rage, rage against the dying of the light." ~Dylan Thomas

Worn out from the heaviness of it all, Jim leaned back to rest. He no sooner settled in for a moment of peace than his nose started to gush blood. He seemed stable otherwise, but we couldn't get the bleeding to stop, and we did *not* want to go back to the hospital. The nosebleed was the first portent signaling the end game from a body that was being consumed by cancer cells. I called the cancer center for instruction, but the nosebleed started literally one minute after they shut the phones off for the day, so we got bumped to on-call. Rather than wait for someone to call back, I asked my sister Diane to come back to Rochester to help us out. She'd been yo-yoing back and forth between Buffalo and Rochester for the last several days. She arrived in an hour armed with supplies to pack his nose and slow the flow. To our great relief, we were able to get the hemorrhage under control.

Jim's body was changing rapidly. His legs swelled up like parade balloons. His eyes were bulging, and his resting face was without emotion, like the mask of Parkinson's. He reverted to needing the walker, and he seemed not quite himself anymore. Despite his rapidly declining condition, he was determined to have a few last visits. He dug deep, tapping into some crazy kind of Herculean strength to hold the cancer back long enough to carry out his final wishes.

While my husband was demonstrating a bravery that people only write about, I was dithering away, trying to figure out what to do, not yet realizing that *doing* was no longer necessary. Caregivers often have trouble accepting that sitting quietly, listening, and being fully present is the most important support one can provide their dying person. After the freneticism of our six-month cancer battle, it was time for me to lay down my arms. It was time for me to let it be. But I wasn't quite there yet. Two energy currents pulsed through our home. One filled with acceptance and determination to finish life in peace, while the other was laden with static electricity from fear and ignorance. I could not fathom what dying was going to look like. As I talked with Jim, I thought: *How are you going to go from aliving to dying?* This will sound strange, but my mind drifted to Linda McCartney. When she passed away, I remember her obituary reported that two days before she died, she rode her beloved horse. It was as remarkable to me in 1998 as it was in that moment. *How can a person be so alive like that, and then, just, dead?*

Fortunately, bolstered by a sense of purpose, Jim pulled me out of my head by keeping me on task to make his arrangements. He was clear and specific when he asked me to gather our families. Essentially, he wanted me to organize a living wake.

Making meaning

In between summoning family members to our home, I took a moment to post a note on CaringBridge. I thanked friends and family for their support and invited people to share with Jim what was in their hearts over text and email. What followed was a steady flow of the most touching notes I'd ever read in my life. People from near and far shared memories and reflections on their relationship with Jim. They talked about his generous spirit, his easygoing style, his availability to talk when friends needed him, his laughter, kindness, and genuine friendship.

The most moving notes came from the young men who grew up with Jim in their lives. Young men who felt safe and supported in his presence during their formative years opened their hearts to expose a garden of love, respect, gratitude, and sadness. Without hesitation or self-consciousness, eloquent notes came in from cousins, nephews, our sons' friends, and the sons of Jim's friends. The words were poetic, heartfelt, and sincere.

Jim moved a demographic that is repeatedly labeled as unable to communicate emotionally. The vulnerability these guys shared with Jim in his final days was one of the greatest parting gifts he could have received. That his genuine love, affection, hard work, and commitment to family and friendship throughout his life had an impact on a generation of people who were caught in the maelstrom of a once-in-a-lifetime pandemic and staggering socio-political chaos was a legacy to be proud of.

Around two o'clock on Saturday, July 18th, before the family visits started, a young woman showed up. She looked apprehensive as she came into my house and announced she was from palliative care. Relieved, I started asking all my care questions, but she stopped me mid-sentence to explain that she was the intake person, not a care nurse. What? What does that mean? She explained she was only there to fill out paperwork on the patient *for* the care nurse. When I led her upstairs to see Jim, she looked downright fearful. I couldn't tell if it was because she wasn't used to coming into someone's home, or because she didn't know how to talk to a dying person. I gave her a seat across from Jim who was lying in bed. She proceeded to ask all the "name, rank and serial number" questions. Are you fucking kidding me? Clearly, we needed some assistance. She told me no one was coming to help me until Monday. *Fuck sake.*

After the "intake person" left, the boys and I helped Jim get dressed and moved him downstairs so he could receive people in the living room. Jim's immediate family was on their way over for the first round of visits. Ever the consummate host, he greeted his family with warm, welcoming embraces, as if this was just another normal party we were throwing. One could have easily been swept up in the notion of normalcy if it wasn't for Jim's terrible physical appearance. Only fourteen days away from his fifty-seventh birthday, he looked like a frail old man. His skin clung to his bald skull as if it were shrink-wrapped, emphasizing his bulging eyes. Jim's smile was from the heart, but his body wasn't cooperating. The muscles in his face were taut, making his smile look more like a pained grimace. Though the majority of his body was sickly skinny, his legs were freakishly large from swelling. This grim combination made Jim look like a goblin from a fantasy fiction novel. Covid kept his family away during the bone marrow transplant recovery process, so it was a complete and utter shock for them to see how he'd declined in three short months. Still, they all did an adequate job of hiding their horror at being met by a man who was unrecognizable. The Barberos are a family of talkers, so it wasn't hard for them to make conversation. They pressed past their initial shock and chatted about this and that, trying to enjoy their last gathering together as best they could.

Throughout the visit, his mother tried to stifle her tears. I'm mad at myself for creating an atmosphere that inhibited her. I was afraid if she cried inconsolably, then Jim would get upset and cry, and I guess I didn't know what to do with that. In hindsight, everyone should have cried their eyes out with Jim, because deep sadness was the right feeling to have. Otherwise, we were all being emotionally dishonest.

Though the visit was pretty short by Barbero standards, Jim was getting tired, so we gathered for one last family photo. That seems macabre, but it was important for me to have it. I can't explain why. Maybe another way to bear witness to an important life that mattered to me and so many others. When his family left, there were a lot of "I love you's," but no "goodbyes." No one could bring themselves to say it.

It was amazing how Jim perked up for his final visits. The next day he received my family at the dining room table with the same enthusiasm as the day before. Jim told my parents he wasn't afraid of dying, but he wanted to go quickly and painlessly. Again, I tried to dilute the seriousness of what he was saying in a *Let's keep it light for company* kind of way. *Ack! Shut up Jennifer! It's too late to shield anyone from this painful reality. And why would you want to?*

That evening, we welcomed two of Jim's closest friends. As the sun set, we brought him out back in a wheelchair so we could visit next to our vegetable garden. While we chatted, Jim could look around and take stock and pride in all the work he'd done over the years to make our house a home. The little stick of a cherry tree Jim planted to commemorate Giacomo's birth was now taller than the house. We had a healthy thicket of heirloom concord grapes Jim nurtured from the cuttings a neighbor gave us when we first moved in. They grew over a pergola Jim built using salvaged pillars from a neighbor's porch reconstruction. The combination of shade from the cherry tree and grape vines kept us cool in the summers as we sat on the slate patio he built. We could admire the garage roof Jim restored with Gianni and the interesting "citybilly" cover Jim built around our grill to keep us dry while cooking in inclement weather. The vegetable garden itself would have made our Italian ancestors proud. Over the years, the garden took many shapes and forms, giving us an annual opportunity to try different plants, methods, and designs. All of this was contained by the fence Jim installed when we adopted our first German Shepherd, Roxy.

We had a front row seat to the circle of life that played out in our yard for 23 years. Now, it was like we were looking into an infinity mirror as Jim's life was about to end. In our brief time in the yard that evening, sadness was joined by awe at the wonder and mystery of life.

Between the visits, Jim was uncomfortable and restless. Once I realized the Saturday palliative lady wasn't going to help us, I called the cancer center and left messages with anyone who would listen. We needed help. Monday came and the cancer center called me to say I could bring Jim in for a blood transfusion to see if that would provide him some comfort. While there, a number of people came in to talk to us. Mostly they came in to say goodbye. It was tender and kind. Still, no one pulled me aside and told me what to expect and what to do.

The transfusion didn't provide any relief. Medical interventions no longer acted as a speed bump to the cancer that was swarming my husband's insides. It was time to switch over to hospice care. The one thing I remember Dr. Wonderful telling us was that we could switch from palliative to hospice at any time. At this point in our story, it won't shock you to learn that that was not the case. They sent us home again with no end-of-life instructions. After we got back from the transfusion center, an actual palliative home nurse came to see Jim. He informed us that they couldn't provide hospice care until Thursday. *Oh my God! Are you kidding me?*

We continued with the final visits. That afternoon we welcomed Jim's band members; he wanted to see his second family one last time. After they left, the boys and I helped Jim up the stairs. His physical condition was declining rapidly. Part way up, he told us this would be the last time we'd have to help him because he wouldn't be coming back down again. The weight of his words settled on us like a millstone.

Later that afternoon, my sister Robin and her family made it in from Pittsburgh to say their goodbyes while Jim lay in our bed. That was the last of the visits. He had seen everyone he wanted to see. He gave people the watercolor paintings he wanted them to have. He heard from friends and family how much he meant to them and told them the same back. Throughout this living wake, I was repeatedly surprised by the number of grown men sobbing. My husband was dear to many people. His kindness, empathy, generous spirit, and vulnerability gave other men access to theirs. The loving goodbyes Jim received in return were befitting of a king. The kind of king that was a pauper in the purse but infinitely rich with friendship.

Welcome to our shit show

From Monday into Tuesday, calls were flying around between the cancer center and home care. The same medical professionals who could see with their own eyes that my husband was dying kept scheduling appointments with palliative care well into the future. I'm not sure where Dr. Wonderful was in all of this. After his verbose presentation in the hospital, I never heard from him again. The bone marrow transplant nurse coordinator was our point person for Jim's end-of-life care. Maybe someday someone will explain the wisdom of that staffing decision to me.

While the faceless healthcare administrators were playing hot potato with our case, Jim was becoming exceedingly uncomfortable. He was plagued by a restlessness and irritation that couldn't be assuaged. Lacking appropriate instruction or support, I tried to figure out how to wean him off his prescribed medicines (like the powerful steroid he was on) to see if that was what was causing his agitation. I didn't understand that his restlessness was part of the dying process. That this is what life's offramp looked like. Because we made the choice of going home with palliative care, I was focused on the entirely wrong kind of symptom management. And it wasn't helping my husband one bit. Finally, the transplant nurse coordinator indicated they were able to muster up a hospice nurse to see Jim on Wednesday and gave me a prescription for morphine, but the dosing wasn't high enough, so his agitation continued to escalate. Tuesday night, Jim was up every hour with an unrelenting urge to urinate. The persistent feeling left him uncomfortable and frustrated. His legs were so swollen with fluid, standing to use the urinal was precarious. I'd jump up every time he moved to help him and make sure he didn't fall. He'd lean against the bed to steady himself while I held the urinal for him, but very little, if anything came out. The frustration for Jim was beyond vexing.

Practically delirious from exhaustion myself, I was counting the seconds until the hospice nurse would arrive on Wednesday. I was fully expecting them to show me how to get, and keep, Jim comfortable. By 1 p.m. Wednesday, Jim's agitation started spiraling into delirium. The nurse arrived in the middle of Jim arguing with us because he wanted to use the bathroom. We had the commode set up next to the bed, but he was insisting on walking to the bathroom to use the toilet. He was terribly unsteady; I was terrified he was going to fall so we were preventing him from leaving the room all the while pleading with him to use the commode. His combativeness reached a fevered pitch as he started waving us off and yelling at us in Italian. I can only assume, but in that moment, I think part of his agitation was his reluctance to use the commode in front of his family. His body and mind may have been failing, but his modesty and pride remained intact.

The nurse witnessed the entire ordeal, but didn't provide assistance, instruction, or information about what was happening. Yet another healthcare professional avoiding the responsibility of explaining what dying looked like. She explained that she wasn't a hospice nurse there to help us. She was yet *another* intake nurse, sent to ask the same "name, rank and serial number" questions and to fill out the same paperwork that everyone else filled out a thousand fucking times. She told me her role was to assess the situation and order whatever equipment we needed.

Jim finally gave up fighting with us and sat on the commode to defecate. The explosive elimination reminded me of Giacomo's diaper blow-outs that were legendary at daycare. Loudly percussive, soft, yellow infant-like feces violently ejected out of Jim's body. The elimination was a huge relief to everyone in the room. Once Jim was finished, I cleaned him up and got him settled back into bed while the boys cleaned up everything else. The entire ordeal exhausted all of us. His anger, the arguing in Italian, the physical opposition—it was all too much.

Following that episode, the intake nurse realized she was out of her depth and put my sister on the phone with the director of hospice. They spoke, doctor to doctor. Diane got all the information and instructions we needed to execute Jim's care. The hospice doctor ordered a bunch of medicines, and our sons were dispatched to the pharmacy. Jim was now sitting on the edge of our bed, lucid again, with a look of defeat on his face. With his hands gently resting on my hips, he looked up into my face pleadingly. He wanted a painless, dignified end of life. So far, we weren't on track to make that happen. The look of sadness in his eyes created a permanent wound in my heart. I was failing at this miserably. Worn out from his "rage against the dying of the light," episode, he was past ready to go gently. He opened his mouth like a hungry baby bird, and I gave him a dose of morphine to settle him down and tucked him into bed where he drifted off to sleep.

Shell-shocked from the pandemonium, I sat down to catch my breath. Trepidation vibrated in my bones as the unknown rapidly unfolded before me. We didn't know if he was going to wake up again possessed by the same ferocity he displayed during the commode episode. And if he did, I knew I was at the end of my ability to manage him physically. The kids didn't want round two either, but we were all torn. We desperately wanted to care for Jim at home, but we were afraid we weren't capable of doing it.

Jolted into action by the literal shit storm she walked into, the nurse called the hospital to check and see if there was a hospice bed available. She reported that there was a bed, but we needed to decide immediately if we were going to take it. Knowing we had another option to make sure Jim was properly cared for in the event he woke up swinging again acted as a pressure release valve.

The boys and I took a moment to discuss the matter privately. There were several factors to consider. First, every one of us, including Jim, hated the hospital. All of us wanted to provide him the peace and comfort of our home in his last days. Then, the reality of the parade of emergency personnel required to transfer Jim to the hospital was more than any of our nerves could take. Lastly, there was the added burden that continued to weigh us down throughout our cancer odyssey: Covid. The hospital regulations would have prevented all of us from being together in Jim's final hours.

Our fears of having to forcefully contain him again and possibly hurting him, sparking the final decline, fueled our hesitation to keep him home. But things had changed for the better in a short period of time. We now had all the prescriptions we needed, and my sister had received thorough instructions from the hospice director on how to administer them to keep Jim comfortable. Now that he was settled, caring for him seemed less harrowing. We were unanimous in forgoing hospital hospice and opted instead to stay put.

Once we confirmed our choice, the nurse went back to grilling me with a battery of questions. I answered her robotically while I watched my husband sleep. She paused in the middle of her questions, as if she finally realized what was happening, and went off script. I guess maybe to seem more relatable, she started asking me about our sons. I was telling her how hard it was for them to watch their father suffer. Instead of taking time to explain body systems and what to expect from here on out, she chose to say one of the most ridiculous things I'd ever heard: "Well, you never know. Maybe because of this, one of your sons will discover the cure for cancer." Despite my fast-approaching catatonic state, I had to stifle myself from releasing a bitter laugh in her face. *What the fuck are you talking about?!* I thought. *How is that supposed to comfort me right now? My kids discovering a cure for cancer isn't going to help us right now. And, we're artists for God's sake! Why would you say something so stupid?* Her words were insensitive, and uninformed, reflecting the fact that she had no idea what she was talking about. So it's okay that my husband is dying if one of our sons becomes a doctor? It's like a line she heard out of a movie. My urge to laugh was quickly replaced with disgust. Her ludicrous reflection revealed that the agency sent over someone completely unqualified to be in this situation. It was like I was talking to a five-year-old. I barely remember finishing the questionnaire or her packing up and leaving.

CHAPTER TWENTY-ONE

The Dimming of the Day

As the sun set, we all milled about the house not really knowing what to do with ourselves while Jim slept. At nine o'clock, my sister came upstairs to tell me that there was a delivery man at my door. *What now?* I thought. Turns out, the intake nurse ordered a bunch of stuff for us—probably because she didn't know what else to do. I went downstairs to find a short, portly man standing in my foyer next to an oxygen machine. "What am I supposed to do with that?" I asked Diane. She went with "It can't hurt." so I accepted the delivery. But before he could set everything up, he needed me to sign my name in about 80 places on a stack of papers as thick as *War and Peace*. I have no idea what I authorized. For all I knew, I accepted a pony along with the oxygen machine.

Once he was satisfied that I'd signed every single piece of paper in his possession, he asked where the patient was. I told him he was upstairs. Not a good answer, judging by the look on his face. Clearly, this guy was in no shape to be carrying something this heavy around. Gianni offered to help him with the machine, but the man declined and said he could do it. He got to the landing and had to take a break. He was huffing and puffing and sweating up a storm. I regretted removing Jim's break chair. He lugged it up the final five stairs and wheeled it into our bedroom. Well, I guess this man didn't realize that he was going to come face to face with a dying person. He was trying hard not to freak out. I couldn't distinguish whether he was sweating from exertion or fear. The dude was drenched. He launched into a speed version of how to use the machine, finishing his litany with a question about what length of hose I would need. I can't remember what I said. All I remember is the response I wanted to give: *I don't fucking know. Everybody, including you, wants you to go. For the love of God, do us all a solid, and please leave.* He hightailed it outta there as if we were all zombies about to eat his face. I never saw a fat guy move so fast.

As soon as the smoke from his exit trail dissipated, Diane leaned over to me and said: "Well, I guess Paul Blart doesn't like dead people." We had a good chuckle over the latest in the cascade of absurdities surrounding Jim's end of life. Aside from that interruption, our day seamlessly melted into night. The boys set up a television in our bedroom so we could huddle around Jim and watch a show together. The oxygen machine was humming along, as the telltale death rattle added a percussive component to Jim's breathing. We chose to watch a comedy about vampires. Odd choice I suppose, but I don't think any of us were actually watching anything. After a couple episodes, we shut the TV off and everyone crawled off to their nests, alone with their deep sadness and fear.

The thinking light

Like a child, I get wound up before I fall asleep at night. My memories of being amped up at bed time go as far back as grade school. My younger sister Robin and I would tell silly jokes and talk smack in the dark, making each other laugh until our gas tanks were empty enough to allow sleep to take over. Maturity never leveled my propensity to process the day's events through a final burst of energy at bedtime. Many a night, I would subject Jim to my nonsense. I'd perform silly bedtime dances to made-up songs, or I'd jump into bed next to him and chatter away about life, the universe, and everything. Sometimes he'd laugh and marvel at what a whacko he married. Other times, he'd get annoyed and tell me to shut the hell up and go to sleep.

We had a nightstand on my side of the bed where our alarm clock and lamp lived. Jim referred to the lamp as my "thinking light," because I'd keep that light on while I chattered away. If I needed to spare my husband the running of my mouth, I'd stare at the ceiling while my thoughts chased each other around in my brain like chipmunks. Eventually, he'd tell me I was burning a hole in the ceiling with my laser focused eyes, and it was time to turn the "thinking light" off, which I would dutifully do, then snuggle up next to him, take his hand in mine, and fall asleep.

When Jim got home from our first tour in the hospital, I retired my thinking light in favor of nightlights. They cast enough light to help us find our way around medical equipment and medicines during Jim's restless nights, but not too much as to disturb his sleep. Entering into what turned out to be our last silent night together, I extinguished the thinking light, allowing the warm glow from the night light to create a reverent atmosphere in what was now a holy space.

Jim was laying on his back, unmoving, while I curled up next to him in the fetal position, holding his hand and listening to his rattly breathing. Diane came in throughout the night on schedule to administer the hospice medicines, then crept back across the hall to her temporary quarters. At one point in the middle of the night, I felt Jim scoop my hand in his. Not a big movement, but enough for me to know it was intentional.

Shortly past 4 a.m., I awoke to Jim's changed breathing pattern. The shallow, rhythmic breath that lulled me to sleep had become short and rapid, almost like panting. His eyes were wide open, fixed, and unflinching. Now *he* was the one staring at the ceiling. His body was rigid and he looked frightened to me. I turned on the thinking light and slowly waved my hand in front of his eyes, but they didn't track. Nor did he respond to my touch or my voice. Rather than call for anyone, I cozied even closer. I knew this was the end and didn't want to disturb this sacred moment.

While Jim worked at dying, I gently whispered in his ear. I told him how much I loved him; how much we all loved him and that we were going to miss him very much. Though I instinctively knew that there was nothing left to do to help him, my impulse to provide comfort wasn't satisfied with taking a seat and allowing this organic process to unfold without some intervention. Feeling a little desperate, as I repeated my professions of love, I decided to add in words about the old-fashioned God we learned about in our Catholic upbringing. I clumsily said something about how God loved him and was waiting for him. Funny enough, my words caused *more* agitation. He actually started choking. Even in dying, my husband could recognize disingenuous words. I quickly went back to telling him how much I loved him while gently stroking his cheek. With authenticity restored, his choking stopped and he relaxed back into a rhythmic panting. Cuddling up even closer, tears stung my eyes as sorrow squeezed my voice when I whispered to him that it was ok for him to go. That we would miss him terribly, but it was okay to let go.

The quickening is described as the moment a pregnant woman feels her baby move for the first time. Some say it's the point in fetal development when the cell cluster becomes a human being. Perhaps when they receive their soul. As the sun set on Jim's life, it seemed he was experiencing a version of the quickening. His body struggled with transition, much like a baby laboring to be expunged from its mother's womb.

The tension caused by life and death pulling away from each other wracked my husband's body. I wondered if it was fear I saw in his eyes, or concentration on the task at hand. I'd like to think that after six months, Jim was finally in charge. Rather than quietly melting into a decrescendo, I imagine his spirit queuing a lively fanfare preceding his arrival into the next realm. All I needed to do was stay in the moment. For better or for worse. In sickness and in health. Until death do us part.

Over the arc of Jim's illness, we engaged in an emotional clutching of one another. That desperation dissipated in our last moment of intimacy. Before a new day dawned, in the quiet of our marital bed, we knew it was time to honor our love with release. Jim's labored breathing ceased, and with one last deep inhale, our time to let go was upon us. The peace of eternity moved through us on the breath of his final exhale, and, in so moving, Jim passed away, taking my fear of death with him. His final gift.

Epilogue

Three years have passed since we lost Jim in the cancer battle, and the world is a very different place. The global pandemic officially came to an end. My family expanded our menagerie by adopting a puppy. With purpose and determination, Giacomo and Gianni flew the coop to opposite corners of the country to pursue their careers in the arts. The youth of America escalated their hijinks from eating Tide Pods to stealing Kias while "we the people" traded in a president who kept our Cortisol levels revving at an all-time high for an elderly man with whom we feel safe enough to take a nap without worrying about whether or not we're going to wake up to Armageddon. Yes, in three years, many things have changed, with the exception of one: Jim suffered, died, and was buried. That cold, hard fact remains the same no matter how hard I tried to reach beyond my mortal coil to create a literary resurrection.

People look to me with hopeful eyes when they ask me if writing our story has helped me to heal. I'm sorry to say that my answer doesn't include a feel-good Hollywood ending. This book has helped me process the trauma of our cancer experience. However, with regard to healing, I regret to report that there is no healing. There's only learning to live with a wounded soul.

With his final breath, Jim did take away my fear of death. But the yin to that yang has been my daily struggle to find the courage to live without him. Though I work, visit with friends and family, laugh, cry, eat, and sleep fine, there's a faint numbness tamping down my emotions leaving me unable to fully experience joy or happiness the way I used to. It's like the feeling I have in my face when the Novocaine hasn't completely worn off after dental surgery, but it's throughout my psyche. The numbness doesn't trouble me because the energy that would normally feed heights of joy has been redirected to my emotional growth in other areas. I've experienced a deeper level of sadness that I didn't know was possible. But all the tears that I cry water the compost growing in the dead spot left behind by my beloved's departure, and compassion and empathy for the human condition are growing beautifully.

It's my larger capacity for compassion that draws me to a type of work that makes most people recoil, and that is hospice care. My hands used to help people grow their power and wealth. Now, I've turned my talents to helping humans access the assets within themselves, and to find the strength to persevere in what may feel like their darkest hours. It's an honor to be with people at end of life. The dying hold a holy space that should be approached with an abundance of love, respect and silent witness. Death is as great a miracle as birth and deserves the same support and attention that families receive when they welcome a new one into the world. It is in these spaces where I feel whole and content. So much so that I've decided to go back to school to get my Masters in mental health counseling. I'd like to deepen my engagement with patients and families struggling with chronic and terminal illness. I can think of no better way to honor my husband than to become part of the patient care solution.

As a natural-born advocate, it's important to me that this book be used as an education tool for healthcare providers, and a resource for patients, and patient families. The issues we faced throughout Jim's short illness and death are not unique to us. I'm hoping our story can shed light on some of the gaps in the system and provide comfort to those feeling alone as they face a life-altering illness.

If you find yourself caught up in the US healthcare industry, it's important to be mindful of the inherent conflicts born of this profit-driven system. *Patient-Centered Care* doesn't exist for those who can't afford it. And it's limited by what is reimbursable for those who can. Compassionate humans who work in healthcare learn to live with this dichotomy, but I don't think it's easy for them.

You may have been confused by my mercurial reflections on who I liked or disliked on our care teams. That ambiguity was intentional and indicative of the inherent conflict I'm talking about. In my opinion, it's a bad system that breeds distrust and creates an *us vs. them* dynamic out of the patient / care provider relationship. But it's a system powered by all kinds of people. So how do we, in our own way, work compassionately within a system that stokes fear while we're in a vulnerable state? Well, Jesuit priest Father Greg Boyle says we all belong to each other. If you carry that sentiment in your heart, you'll find that loving feels so much better than hating, and grace and compassion are much more fulfilling and freeing than judgment and criticism. It's hard, but if you can wrap those notions around you while under duress, you may find comfort, protection, and a pathway to patient / provider collaboration.

Three years out, with those ideas in my heart and on my mind, I can safely say to all the people I wanted to punch in the face, I'd like to give you a hug. We all matter, so take care of yourselves and one another.

Thank you for spending your precious time with us. With love and gratitude- Jennifer

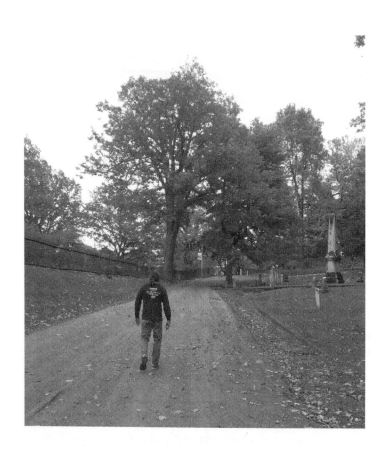

Acknowledgements

In telling the story of what happened to us during Jim's cancer life, I share many of my deepest thoughts and feelings as they happened. There were instances throughout our journey that were irritating, upsetting and downright infuriating. I decided not to eliminate or dilute them. Staying close to the emotions has helped me process my grief and understand how to direct my anger. In the end, the main offender was cancer.

I did not use the names of our care professionals, recognizing that, in the midst of our cancel culture, using names may cause harm and that most definitely is not my intent. I respected and appreciated most of our caregivers. For those I didn't, well, that doesn't define who they are as professionals or as people. It's just one family's experience at a point in time.

To all our doctors, nurses and health care professionals, thank you for taking care of Jim to the best of your abilities. My husband had a nasty disease. With intention and genuine care, you did everything you could to help him fight it off. We are particularly grateful to the outstanding nurses at the Wilmot Cancer Center. You are a remarkable team of talented and compassionate professionals.

Words alone can't convey how deeply grateful I am to my editors. My learning curve as a first-time author, combined with the agony of reliving our story repeatedly, made this an incredibly difficult project. Molly Clifford, Scott Cole, Aaron DeBee, Ellen Leverich, Amy Levey, Wendy Low, and Jason Yungbluth, your patience, encouragement and excellent reviews of my work were instrumental in helping me get my story over the finish line. I will be forever grateful to you for lending your expertise and attention to detail while giving space to my grieving brain.

I am fortunate to be flush with the most important natural resource known to humans: friends. There are so many beautiful people in my life who supported me and encouraged me while I worked on this project. To all of you, thank you for your friendship, support and love. No doubt, it's what carried me through as I labored over this important work.

To the folks on the front lines: My mom, dad and siblings–Sam, Diane, Mark, Robin–and their families; my mother-in-law Rose and the Barbero clan; Molly, Ellen, Christine, Jane, Peg and Fran, Beth, Christopher and Liam, Elissa, Kate, Carl, Jennifer, Molly & Darlene, Josh and Lori, Jill, Mardi, Amy and "John", Amy and Michael, my friends at Pat's Coffee Mug, Kevin (and Spatz and Smoke), the gang at Enright's, Kristin and my Isaiah House family, Kauser Ahmed and Chris and my process group peeps. Thank you for answering my random phone calls and texts, for talking me through my writer's block, providing counsel, or just holding space for me.

My sons gave great guidance, advice and <ahem> *opinions* that I needed to hear. Thank you, Giacomo and Gianni, for collaborating with me, and taking risks to tolerate some pain in order to support my work. It is better because of your input.

Lastly, I would be remiss if I didn't acknowledge my incredibly self-centered, furry support team: Buster, Lucy, Skitchey and Vera. They did an excellent job of sitting on my keyboard, chewing my pens and barfing on my rough drafts. Thank you for making sure I got out of bed.

ABOUT THE AUTHOR

Born and raised in Buffalo, NY (*Go Bills!*), Jennifer Sanfilippo, MBA, enjoyed a robust career as a trusted executive advisor and political strategist. She brought her thoughtful, strategic sensibilities first to the public sector, advising members of Congress, governors, mayors and senior staffers at the federal, state and local levels. Mid-career, she transitioned to the private sector, advising senior executives at several financial institutions in New York State. Since Jim's passing, Jennifer has turned her attention to providing support and counsel to those facing major life transitions, and facilitating end-of-life conversations. She is the delighted mother of two magnificent young men, and lives in comfortable co-dependence with her three cats in Rochester, NY.

Visit Jennifer's website at www.jennifer-sanfilippo.com for more information and links to resources on end-of-life care, leukemia and other related areas of interest.

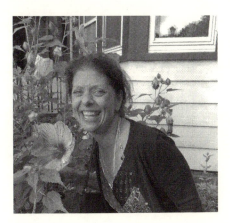

Made in the USA
Middletown, DE
26 March 2024

51864010R00151